HEALTH&WEIGHT-LOSS
BREAKTHROUGHS 2011

HEALTH&WEIGHT-LOSS
BREAKTHROUGHS 2011

SMART STRATEGIES TO FEEL YOUNG AND LOOK GREAT

FROM THE EDITORS OF **Prevention**.

RODALE

© 2011 by Rodale Inc.

Photo credits are on page 351.

ISBN 13: 978-1-60529-171-0

2 4 6 8 10 9 7 5 3 1 hardcover

We inspire and enable people to improve their lives and the world around them

For more of our products visit **rodalestore.com** or call 800-848-4735

CONTENTS

PART 3
FITNESS MOVES

PART 4
NUTRITION NEWS

PART 5
MIND MATTERS

PART 6
BEAUTY BASICS

INTRODUCTION

YOU-ONLY HEALTHIER! That's what this book offers. Here are tips and tricks to help you look younger, feel better, and be the best you ever! You hold in your hand a collection of all the newest breakthroughs and most recent studies to help you to enhance your health and improve your life.

Part 1: Health Breakthroughs highlights the amazing innovations that can protect your heart, fight cancer, save you from Alzheimer's, and improve the way you feel each and every day. You'll learn how to recognize the surprising signs you'll live to 100, how to stay flu-free without becoming obsessive about disinfecting everything, and how to separate fact from fiction about home DNA testing.

Part 2: Weight-Loss Wisdom offers the latest information about dropping pounds. Discover little-known diet saboteurs and how to fight them, find some new flips for weight loss, and shed pounds quickly with our weight-loss plans.

In addition, we've included a Bonus Weight-Loss Cookbook. We love the Chocolate-Stuffed French Toast, Lemon-Blueberry Buttermilk Muffins, Cinnamon Sweet Potatoes with Vanilla, Gingered Chicken and Greens Stir-Fry, and Pumpkin Pecan Pie—and we bet your family will, too.

You'll be inspired to move more by Part 3: Fitness Moves. Your body is craving the workouts here, including the essential over-40 workout and the Yes-You-Can-Run Plan. Plus, you'll mistake-proof your exercise routine with the surprising workout blunders we've uncovered here.

In Part 4: Nutrition News, you'll learn how to eat better than ever with food combos that really add up. Then we'll detail key information about three nutrition news stories you don't want to miss; high fructose corn syrup, omega-3 fatty acids, and the superbug in your supermarket.

Boost your mental well-being with the new strategies and innovations in Part 5: Mind Matters. You can make your home a haven, find seven ways to boost your brainpower, get energy for life, and enjoy better sleep.

In Part 6: Beauty Basics, we've collected our favorite tips and tricks to turn back time. Here's how to get great skin, whether you have a day, a week, or a month. You'll learn the ABCs of beautiful skin. Save money and time with hair color that lasts. And get ready to give up your excuses, because we've found sunscreens you'll love to wear.

We've filled this book with the latest and greatest health and weight-loss news and information. Here's to your health and happiness!

Part 1

HEALTH
Breakthroughs

CHAPTER 1

TOP MEDICAL Breakthroughs

Fight cancer, prevent a heart attack, protect your brain from Alzheimer's disease, and more.

These remarkable innovations promise to revolutionize the way doctors prevent, diagnose, and treat common conditions and diseases. Plus, they can help you take control of your own health and well-being.

BREAKTHROUGH THAT COULD PREVENT AND TREAT CANCER NATURALLY

In 2009, the American College of Sports Medicine (ACSM) certified its first group of cancer exercise trainers. The new program reflects fresh thinking about the way physical activity can help prevent and treat cancer. "Oncologists who once thought cancer patients should take it easy are beginning to prescribe exercise as a form of medicine," says exercise physiologist Richard Cotton, ACSM's national director of certification and registry programs.

Research finds that exercise can lower recurrence rates and boost survival among women who have had cancer. One review found that moderate activity,

THE BUILDING BLOCKS OF A BREAKTHROUGH

Most advances don't come from sudden flashes of insight but from small steps that add up to giant leaps. Here are some seemingly minor developments with big implications.

Instant Immunity

SMALL STEP: Scientists at the Scripps Research Institute have developed a vaccination technique that produces an immune response using engineered chemical reactions instead of inactive germs or other disease-causing agents.

GIANT LEAP: Vaccines could work almost immediately instead of over the weeks that many require to become effective. First an injected chemical primes the immune system for a fight; then specially designed molecules bind to a specific target and tell the altered immune cells where to attack.

"In addition to rapidly protecting you from getting sick, instant immunity would slow the spread of virulent diseases like the flu," says Scripps professor Carlos Barbas III, PhD.

A Weapon against the Worst Cancers

SMALL STEP: A new class of drugs, PARP inhibitors, has been shown to block specific enzymes in stubborn cancer cells that repair their own DNA damage.

such as brisk walking 3 hours a week, reduced breast and colon cancer deaths by about 50 percent.

Bottom line. Exercise is a potent weapon against the disease both before and after diagnosis.

BREAKTHROUGH THAT COULD THIN BLOOD MORE SAFELY

For decades, the blood thinner of choice for people at high risk of stroke has been warfarin (Coumadin), which is a tricky drug that doctors must monitor

GIANT LEAP: "Cancer cells that can't repair DNA damage caused by chemo die more easily," says Ernest T. Hawk, MD, MPH, vice president for Cancer Prevention and Population Science at the University of Texas M. D. Anderson Cancer Center. In studies, PARP inhibitors have proved effective against aggressive, difficult-to-treat cases of breast cancer, including genetic disease and tumors that resist chemotherapy. Importantly, when combined with chemo, PARP treatment typically adds few side effects, because normal cells stay healthy by using other backup repair enzymes that cancer cells lack.

"This is an entirely new approach to fighting some of our worst diseases, and it has the potential to save thousands of lives," says Dr. Hawk.

Hope for a Cancer Vaccine

SMALL STEP: In a study at M. D. Anderson, an experimental cancer vaccine combined with the immunotherapy drug Interleukin-2 shrank tumors in 22 percent of people with advanced melanoma, which is one of the most lethal cancers, and improved their survival by 5 months.

GIANT LEAP: The study marks one of the first successful trials of a therapeutic cancer vaccine after decades of research.

"People who benefited saw their tumors shrink by half or more," says Dr. Hawk. "We haven't seen that before in real people, only in lab dishes." Giving the vaccine to patients in early stages should boost survival even more, he says.

carefully—often with weekly tests—because it interacts with other medications and increases the risk of bleeding.

Now, a new drug called dabigatran prevents more strokes with less bleeding than warfarin, according to a study of 18,113 people with atrial fibrillation, a key risk factor for stroke. The study, published in the *New England Journal of Medicine*, marks the first time in more than 50 years that a new blood thinner has been found that is considered more effective than the existing gold standard, says study leader Stuart Connolly, MD, director of the Division of Cardiology at McMaster University in Ontario.

"It's a triple win, because the new drug is also easier to use," he says. "It doesn't interact with many other medications, so you don't need to test and adjust the dose constantly."

Dabigatran is available as Pradaxa in Canada and Europe; FDA approval is pending.

BREAKTHROUGH THAT MIGHT PROTECT THE WORLD AGAINST HIV

Researchers at the International AIDS Vaccine Initiative and The Scripps Research Institute in La Jolla, California, have discovered two new antibodies—produced by a minority of people—that offer hope for an HIV vaccine. Because the new antibodies are "broadly neutralizing," they cripple many different strains of the deadly virus.

Four other broadly neutralizing antibodies are known to exist, but the new weapons are more potent, latch on to their targets more easily, and are the first to have been isolated from people in the developing world, where 95 percent of new AIDS cases occur. Researchers are now working on developing an active ingredient to put into a vaccine that would stimulate the production of these antibodies.

BREAKTHROUGH THAT COULD PREVENT HEART ATTACKS IN HIGH-RISK PATIENTS

Omega-3 fatty acids have been upgraded from nutritional supplement to bona fide heart medicine: Lovaza, a prescription medication, purifies and concentrates 3 to 4 times more EPA and DHA into pills than fish oil capsules contain and is approved by the FDA to treat high triglycerides. Now a 2009 review of four major studies (many using Lovaza) shows that omega-3s help treat the highest-risk heart patients—those who have had a heart attack or heart failure.

"These patients were already being vigorously treated with other therapies, and omega-3s lowered their risks even more," says Carl Lavie, MD, medical director of cardiac rehabilitation and prevention at the John Ochsner Heart and Vascular Institute in New Orleans.

(continued on page 8)

BREAKTHROUGHS CLOSE TO HOME

We asked *Prevention*'s partners, *The Doctors,* hosts of the eponymous CBS hit show: What innovation has changed how you help patients or how they help themselves?

Omega-3s for Brain Health

In addition to their anti-inflammatory benefits for adults, omega-3s improve babies' brain development and immunity. Now the fatty acids are routinely added to formula and benefit the millions of infants who can't breast-feed. I try to ensure that all my patients (and their parents!) take a supplement.
—Pediatrician Jim Sears, MD

Easier, More Effective CPR

Giving only chest compressions—without mouth-to-mouth—produces a better outcome for people in cardiac arrest. Enough oxygen remains in the blood, so a rescuer should focus only on compressions. This is huge: Each minute that passes before resuscitation begins decreases survival by 10 percent.
—ER physician Travis Stork, MD

HPV Testing and Vaccine

HPV testing is a way of identifying which women are at high risk for cervical cancer so we can screen them more frequently with Pap tests and pick up precursors (abnormal cell changes) sooner, and thus save more women's lives.
—Ob-gyn Lisa Masterson, MD

Safer Skin Protection

With the new fractional lasers, we can more effectively fight wrinkles and brown spots without older lasers' potential side effects, like redness. As a bonus, people will see a reduction in actinic keratoses (lesions that are a precursor to cancer).
—Plastic surgeon Drew Ordon, MD

His review also found that EPA and DHA lower risks of atrial fibrillation and atherosclerosis.

"Yet few doctors seem to realize there's so much impressive evidence supporting omega-3s for cardiovascular protection," he says. His review in the *Journal of the American College of Cardiology* recommends at least 800 to 1,000 milligrams of EPA and DHA combined per day for heart patients, which is an amount many experts recommend for healthy people, too.

BREAKTHROUGH THAT CAN PREDICT A HEART ATTACK OR STROKE

People with high blood pressure or cholesterol are at increased risk of heart attack, but doctors haven't been able to predict who among that group is most likely to have one. Now, a device that clips onto your finger can tell by sensing lack of elasticity in the lining of your blood vessel, a condition called endothelial dysfunction.

"A poor score is a stronger warning than the usual risk factors because it indicates that cardiovascular disease has already begun, but at an early stage when you can more easily control your risks," says Amir Lerman, MD, a cardiologist at the Mayo Clinic in Rochester, Minnesota.

The device, called the EndoPAT, has been FDA-approved since 2003, but a new 8-year study by Dr. Lerman and his colleagues shows that half of people whose scores indicate endothelial dysfunction go on to have a heart attack or stroke, proving that the test is a powerful forecaster of individual risk. A similar system called Vendys is also available.

"It's an extremely important test," says Dr. Lerman, "especially for women, who are more prone to have endothelial dysfunction without other risk factors."

BREAKTHROUGH THAT COULD LEAD TO A CURE FOR ALZHEIMER'S DISEASE

A reliable test for Alzheimer's disease has never existed, but recently, multiple labs around the country broke through the diagnosis barrier. A new method of analyzing MRI images developed at the Mayo Clinic pinpoints changes in the brain with up to 80 percent accuracy. At UCLA, researchers have developed a blood test for AD. But the most accurate and promising technique is a skin test developed at the Blanchette Rockefeller Neurosciences Institute at West Virginia University: With the prick of a finger, it detects defective enzymes involved with memory function that are found in both brain and skin cells.

Test results proved 98 percent accurate at detecting Alzheimer's disease, says Daniel Alkon, MD, the institute's scientific director. Even more remarkable: The researchers discovered that low doses of the chemotherapy drug bryostatin reactivate the defective enzymes.

"We can actually rewire broken connections in the brain and restore memory," says Dr. Alkon. "That's extraordinarily exciting because it could be used to reverse the dreadful consequences of many brain diseases."

CHAPTER 2

Health Lessons STRAIGHT from the Lab

You won't believe the lengths to which researchers go to test their ingenious cures for achy feet, insomnia, and ho-hum sex. Here are their hot-off-the-petri-dish tips.

Doctors no doubt have plenty of great tips and advice on living a healthier, happier life, but much of their wisdom actually comes from the research results of veteran laboratory scientists and researchers. So why not cut out the middlemen (or women)? Here are some surprising lessons directly from the experts who have performed cutting-edge studies. Use their knowledge today to prevent illness, improve your sex life, sleep more soundly, and much more.

FOOT LAB

The researcher: Charles Lundy, PhD, associate director of foot care research and development at Merck Consumer Care

The Lessons

High-heel insoles ease foot pain. Just ask the guys. "We found a way to design high-heel insoles so that they shift the user's weight back on the heels and off the forefoot—the root of foot pain for many high-heel wearers. Our department at the time was all men; so for the initial tests we conducted, we had some of the male engineers walk around the office in high heels! When we were fairly confident of the design, we did eventually test the insole (Dr. Scholl's For Her High Heel Insoles) with women in clinical studies and found that it made a real difference in making high heels more comfortable."

Good insoles can help all your joints. "We knew insoles and orthotics eased foot pain, but we also proved in clinical studies that they provide pain relief for osteoarthritis in the back, hips, and knees. It was pretty unique to find that something under your foot can help the rest of your body, too."

GERM LAB

The researcher: Charles P. Gerba, PhD, professor and environmental microbiologist, University of Arizona

The Lesson

Use hand sanitizer. "The CDC still pushes hand washing; but in my research, alcohol-based hand sanitizers were actually more effective at reducing bacteria. I personally prefer them to hand washing and usually carry a small bottle around with me. I would do both whenever possible."

HAPPINESS LAB

The researcher: Sonja Lyubomirsky, PhD, professor of psychology, University of California, Riverside

The Lesson

Joy is in your hands. "Nearly half of your happiness is determined by what you do and how you think. That means there are many opportunities to change how you feel. I had one student who was paralyzed in an accident and been hospitalized for months, yet his first emotion was gratitude. Why? He had thought he was going to die, and despite the circumstances, he was grateful he didn't."

SCENT LAB

The researcher: Alan Hirsch, MD, director, Smell & Taste Treatment and Research Foundation

The Lesson

Smelling popcorn can boost your sex life. "Our studies found that men respond to just about any scent with increased penile blood flow. Skip the pricey perfume—it upped blood flow by only 3 percent. The smell of cheese pizza increased it by 5 percent; buttered popcorn, by 9 percent; and the combined scent of lavender and pumpkin pie, a whopping 40 percent."

SKIN LAB

The researcher: Leslie Baumann, MD, professor of dermatology and director of the Division of Cosmetic Dermatology, University of Miami

The Lessons

You can reduce wrinkles. "All of these things may help reduce wrinkles when used regularly: daily sunscreen; topical retinoids like Retin-A; and antioxidants like green tea, vitamin C, and coenzyme Q10, both orally and topically. Your dermatologist can recommend the best dosage of each. Stick with them, as changes don't happen overnight."

Mass-market products are often better than expensive boutique brands. "Mass lines can afford more research and development; they make more money. Among the best: Unilever (which makes Dove and Pond's), L'Oréal (Vichy and La Roche-Posay), and Johnson & Johnson (maker of Neutrogena and Aveeno, which has its own research institute). We did a big study for one of the companies and found that 80 percent of women who followed a skin care regimen with mass-market products showed fewer wrinkles and healthier skin than when they used pricier lines."

SLEEP LAB

The researcher: Patricia Murphy, PhD, clinical researcher and associate director, Laboratory of Human Chronobiology, Weill Cornell Medical College

The Lessons

Nap without guilt. "It's ingrained that dozing during the day may mess up sleep at night, but there's no experimental evidence that says so. We've studied hundreds of napping subjects and found that if the start time is before 2 p.m., you can nap for up to 2 hours without impacting your sleep. So take a nap. It helps your brain recharge."

Try melatonin to sleep better. "We learned this supplement causes body temperature to drop, which is necessary to fall asleep. We're also trying to figure out if it suppresses luteinizing hormone, as higher levels of LH are linked to hot flashes, a common sleep disrupter. If you occasionally have trouble falling asleep, take up to 3 milligrams of melatonin 30 minutes before bed; if you can't stay asleep, look for time-release formulas. Stop taking it and see your doctor if there's no change after 2 months."

ORGANIC LAB

The researcher: Will Daniels, vice president of quality, food safety, and organic integrity, Earthbound Farm

The Lesson

Organic salad greens stay fresher longer than conventional. "We've done extensive side-by-side shelf life testing and found that the quality of organic greens usually lasts longer, meaning you're less likely to throw them out and more likely to use what you paid for. And for greens like baby lettuces and arugula, the price point is now nearly identical to that of conventional versions."

CANCER LAB

The researcher: Mary McHugh, MD, FCAP, Mount Carmel Health System, Columbus, Ohio

The Lesson

Get Pap tests after menopause, too. "The average age for cervical cancer diagnosis isn't 35; it's about 50. Too many women wrongly assume they can stop screenings if their Paps are normal after their childbearing years. I had a 45-year-old patient who skipped her tests for 6 years; in the interim, she developed a high-grade precancerous lesion. It struck me that it was entirely preventable. Keep getting tested as directed by your gynecologist."

FOOD LAB

The researcher: David Nieman, DrPH, Human Performance Laboratory director, Appalachian State University, Boone, North Carolina

The Lesson

Cranberries, green tea, and fish oil can boost your immune system. "I've done about 50 studies on marathon runners—who are 6 times more likely to get sick after a race—and learned that immune cells functioned abnormally for a day or so after extreme exertion. We found that a combination of quercetin (an antioxidant in cranberries and red onions), the green tea extract EGCG, and fish oil helped combat oxidative stress, thus warding off illness. For the average person, a diet rich in fruits, vegetables, green tea, and fish should keep the immune system in shape."

SUPPLEMENTS LAB

The researcher: Tod Cooperman, MD, president, ConsumerLab.com

The Lesson

Buy multivitamins carefully. "The daily value information is incorrect for many nutrients in supplements because the base values haven't been reset by the FDA since 1968. For example, kids' vitamins that claim 100 percent of the DV of vitamin A actually provide 2 to 3 times more than they should and often exceed tolerable intake levels. So ignore the DVs and instead print out the Institute of Medicine's most recent recommendations for nutrients (which you can get at www.consumerlab.com/rdas), and compare the vitamin amounts (typically in international units—IU—and milligrams) to the label on your multi."

WALKING LAB

The researcher: Catrine Tudor-Locke, PhD, walking behavior researcher and associate professor, Pennington Biomedical Research Center

The Lesson

Use a pedometer to count steps, not calories burned. "This is especially true if you're watching your weight. Calculations for energy expenditure are often based on a formula in the pedometer's microprocessor that is not tailored to the individual, so take the calorie number with a big grain of salt. A healthy goal: Work up to 10,000 steps a day."

HAIR LAB

The researcher: Michael Jutt, chemical engineer and director of product development, Frédéric Fekkai & Company

The Lesson

Use conditioner before shampoo on occasion. "While researching an experimental styling material, we discovered that none of our shampoos removed it from hair very well. Some materials from products adhere very tightly to follicles and can build up over time. One day, someone in the lab accidentally used conditioner to wash; she corrected it then by washing with shampoo—and to our surprise, the hair ended up much cleaner. Why does it work? The built-up material gets trapped in the conditioner, then you wash away both with shampoo."

CHAPTER 3

SURPRISING
Signs You'll Live to 100

What you're doing right, and how to do it better, to stay healthy, happy, and strong for years to come

According to the World Bank, the average life expectancy in the United States is 78.4 years. Yet depending on how you live, you might already be extending that. Here's why and how.

You're the life of the party. Outgoing people are 50 percent less likely to develop dementia, according to a recent study of more than 500 men and women age 78 and older from the Karolinska Institutet in Sweden. Participants also described themselves as not easily stressed. Researchers speculate that their more resilient brains might be a result of lower levels of cortisol. Studies show that oversecretion of this "stress hormone" can inhibit brain cells' communication.

Science-backed ways to cut cortisol levels: Meditate, drink black tea, or take a nap.

You run for 40 minutes a day. Scientists in California found that middle-age people who did just that—for a total of about 5 hours a week—lived longer and functioned better physically and cognitively as they got older. The researchers tracked runners and nonrunners for 21 years.

"What surprised us is that the runners didn't just get less heart disease, they also developed fewer cases of cancer, neurologic diseases, and infections," says study author Eliza Chakravarty, MD, an assistant professor of medicine at Stanford School of Medicine. "Aerobic exercise keeps the immune system young."

If you don't like to run, even 20 minutes a day of any activity that leaves you breathless can boost your health, she says.

You like raspberries in your oatmeal. Most Americans eat 14 to 17 grams of fiber per day; add just 10 grams and reduce your risk of dying from heart disease by 17 percent, according to a Netherlands study. Dietary fiber helps reduce total and LDL ("bad") cholesterol, improve insulin sensitivity, and boost weight loss.

One easy fix: Top your oatmeal ($\frac{1}{2}$ cup dry has 4 grams of fiber) with 1 cup of raspberries (8 grams) and you get 12 grams of fiber in just one meal. Other potent fiber-rich foods: $\frac{1}{2}$ cup of 100 percent bran cereal (8.8 grams), $\frac{1}{2}$ cup of cooked lentils (7.8 grams), $\frac{1}{2}$ cup of cooked black beans (7.5 grams), one medium sweet potato (4.8 grams), and one small pear (4.3 grams).

You feel 13 years younger than you are. That's what older people in good health said in a recent survey of more than 500 men and women age 70 and older.

"Feeling youthful is linked to better health and a longer life," says researcher Jacqui Smith, PhD, professor of psychology at the University of Michigan. "It can improve optimism and motivation to overcome challenges, which helps reduce stress and boost your immune system and ultimately lowers your risk of disease."

You embrace techie trends. Learn to Twitter or Skype to help keep brain cells young and healthy, says Sherri Snelling, senior director for Evercare (part of UnitedHealthcare), a group that sponsors an annual poll of US centenarians. Many of the oldest Americans send e-mails, Google lost friends, and even date online. Researchers say that using the latest technology helps keep us mentally spry and also socially engaged.

"Stay connected to friends, family, and current events, and you feel vital and relevant," says Snelling.

You started menopause after age 52. Studies show that naturally experiencing it later can mean an increased life span. One reason: "Women who go through menopause late have a much lower risk of heart disease," says Mary Jane Minkin, MD, clinical professor of obstetrics and gynecology at Yale University School of Medicine.

You make every calorie count. Researchers in St. Louis reported that men and women who limited their daily calories to 1,400 to 2,000 (about 25 percent fewer calories than those who followed a typical 2,000- to 3,000-calorie Western diet) were literally young at heart. Their hearts functioned like those of people 15 years younger.

"It's about not just eating less but getting the most nutrition per calorie," says study author Luigi Fontana, MD, PhD, research assistant professor of medicine at Washington University School of Medicine.

Study subjects stuck to vegetables, whole grains, fat-free milk, and lean meat, and nixed white bread, soda, and candy. If you cut empty calories and eat more nutrient-rich foods, your health will improve, says Dr. Fontana. To find out how many calories you need to maintain a healthy weight, go to www.prevention.com/caloriecalculator.

You had a baby later in life. If you got pregnant naturally after age 44, you're about 15 percent less likely to die during any year after age 50 than your friends who had their babies before age 40, reports a recent University of Utah study.

"If your ovaries are healthy and you are capable of having children at that age, that's a marker that you have genes operating that will help you live longer," says lead researcher Ken R. Smith, PhD, professor of human development at the university.

Your pulse beats 15 times in 15 seconds. That equates to 60 beats per minute, or how many times a healthy heart beats at rest. Most people have resting rates between 60 and 100 bpm, though the closer to the lower end of the spectrum, the healthier. A slower pulse means your heart doesn't have to work as hard and could last longer, says Leslie Cho, MD, director of the Women's Cardiovascular Center at the Cleveland Clinic.

You don't snore. Snoring is a major sign of obstructive sleep apnea (OSA), a disorder that causes you to stop breathing briefly because throat tissue collapses and blocks your airway. In severe cases, this can happen 60 to 70 times per hour. Sleep apnea can cause high blood pressure, memory problems, weight gain, and depression. An 18-year study found that people without OSA were 3 times more likely to live longer than those with severe apnea.

If you snore and have excessive daytime drowsiness or mood changes, talk with your doctor about a referral to a sleep center.

THE NEW MIDDLE AGE

Old thinking: After a certain age, decline is inevitable. New thinking: Smart health habits can extend an active, joyful midlife indefinitely.

Meet the New Middle Age, as personified by a generation of women who are extending the prime of life, with all its rich emotional, intellectual, and spiritual potential, way beyond the short horizons that defined their mothers' middle years. Are you among them? If so, you know that a lengthy, vibrant "second act" rests on two key pillars.

THE FIRST PILLAR: a lifelong commitment to preventive health. This is where we come in. We've sifted through the latest research about how to remain physically strong, ward off diabetes and heart disease, preserve perceptual skills, and bolster an immune-boosting sunny outlook.

THE SECOND PILLAR: an active social life. We're all aware of the protective benefits of emotionally satisfying relationships. Now, new research details the advantages conferred by happy friendships—advantages so powerful they reach even to people on the fringes of those friendships.

We outline the building blocks of the New Middle Age here and show you how to imbue your second act with more personal contentment, joy, and vibrancy than you ever thought possible.

You have a (relatively) flat belly after menopause. Women who are too round in the middle are 20 percent more likely to die sooner (even if their body mass index is normal), according to a National Institute on Aging study. At midlife, it takes more effort to keep waists trim because shifting hormones cause most extra weight to settle in the middle. If your waist measures 35 inches or more (for men, 40 inches or more), try adding strength training, eating a daily serving of omega-3s, and eating more healthy fats.

Building Block: A Strong Heart

It's the engine that drives an active lifestyle, essential to your ability to maintain healthy muscles and bones, a sharp mind, and even an upbeat attitude.

YOUR MOM'S MIDDLE AGE: It was all about cholesterol. If it was normal, she'd ignore it; if it was high, she'd control it with a low-fat diet.

THE NEW MIDDLE AGE: Get a heart scan after menopause. Even women with normal cholesterol levels can have heart disease, so "talk to your doctor about getting a CT coronary artery scan," says Mehdi Razavi, MD, a cardiologist at the Texas Heart Institute. The test, which measures calcium accumulation in arteries (a predictor of heart attack risk), can spot trouble even when other tests, such as those that check cholesterol levels, are normal.

Embrace the Mediterranean diet. Not all heart-healthy diets are created equal. The hands-down winner is the Mediterranean diet, which prevents and even reverses heart disease. People whose diets feature monounsaturated fats from olive or canola oil, nuts, and fish, along with abundant fruits and vegetables, reduced their recurrence of heart problems by 50 to 70 percent, according to the Lyon Diet Heart Study in France.

Building Block: Good Vision

A pair of sharp eyes is key to getting up and down the mountain, so to speak, and reveling in all of nature's glory during the hike. Sadly, age-related macular

(continued)

degeneration (AMD), a disease that damages the retina, eventually threatens the vision of about one-third of people.

YOUR MOM'S MIDDLE AGE: What will be will be. She and her doctors believed that AMD could not be prevented.

THE NEW MIDDLE AGE: See better with supplements. Those with vitamins C and E, beta-carotene, and zinc can slow vision loss by 25 percent in people with early signs of AMD, according to health economist David B. Rein, PhD, a scientist at the research firm RTI International in Research Triangle Park, North Carolina.

Building Block: Comic Relief

A good laugh is one of the easiest and most reliable tools for managing health-debilitating stress.

YOUR MOM'S MIDDLE AGE: She laughed when she felt like it. Experts then thought that a sense of humor was determined only by your genes—you're either cheerful or you're not.

THE NEW MIDDLE AGE: Schedule regular "laughercise." Loma Linda University researcher and associate professor Lee Berk, DrPH, has tested the effects of what he calls "mirthful laughter" by asking volunteers to spend time doing nothing more complicated than watching TV comedies. He found that even anticipating a laugh improves the function of immune-enhancing hormones. Dr. Berk's latest study found that over the course of a year, the levels of good HDL cholesterol in volunteers participating in a mirthful-laughter group jumped 26 percent, while their levels of C-reactive proteins, a measure of inflammation linked to risk of both heart disease and diabetes, dropped 66 percent. "We call it laughercise," he explains, "because the benefits of laughter are so much like those of physical activity."

Building Block: Stable Blood Sugar

For most people, type 2 diabetes is preventable, which means that the associated higher risks of heart attack, circulation problems, and dementia are, too.

YOUR MOM'S MIDDLE AGE: She tried to eat complex carbs—whole grains, nuts, and vegetables, which studies then suggested was the key to preventing diabetes.

THE NEW MIDDLE AGE: Focus more on total calories. "Losing weight if you're overweight is the single most important thing you can do," says William C. Knowler, MD, PhD, MPH, a diabetes researcher with the National Institutes of Health. Osama Hamdy, MD, PhD, of the Joslin Diabetes Center in Boston, says overweight people should shoot to lose about 7 percent of their total body weight: "For most people, that's enough to cut their risk of developing diabetes in half."

Building Block: Keen Hearing

Can you think of a finer late-summer night's activity than attending an outdoor concert on a lush greensward with friends? Unfortunately, one in three Americans has high-frequency hearing loss that diminishes the experience, according to a 2008 report in the *Archives of Internal Medicine.*

YOUR MOM'S MIDDLE AGE: She used earplugs, when she remembered. The only way to protect hearing, she thought, was to avoid sustained loud noises, a leading cause of hearing loss.

THE NEW MIDDLE AGE: Eat your veggies. "We used to think hearing loss occurred when tiny hair cells in the inner ear were torn apart by vibrations from loud noises," explains hearing expert Colleen Le Prell, PhD, an associate professor at the University of Florida. "We now know that part of the problem is the accumulation of free radicals, which are toxic to hair cells." Animal studies show that antioxidants may neutralize free radicals, protecting against both short- and long-term damage. Researchers also just reported that 46 volunteers with age-related hearing loss improved their hearing at all frequencies by taking a combination of antioxidants for 13 weeks. Researchers don't yet know the optimal level or mix of antioxidants for hearing protection. Until they do, take a standard multivitamin and load your plate with antioxidant-rich fruits and vegetables—and, of course, avoid very loud, sustained noises, says Le Prell.

Building Block: Close Connections

They're not only fun to hang around with. Real pals also evoke a host of positive emotions that bolster immunity.

(continued)

YOUR MOM'S MIDDLE AGE: She was all about family. She believed that family and marriage created the most important emotional bonds in a person's life.

THE NEW MIDDLE AGE: Friends save lives. A Harvard School of Public Health study of more than 2,800 women with breast cancer found that those without close friends were 4 times more likely to die than women with 10 or more friends. A Swedish study reports that for heart attack prevention, having friendships is second only to not smoking.

Surrounding yourself with cheerful companions may be especially beneficial. In a surprising report, James H. Fowler, PhD, an associate professor of political science at the University of California, San Diego, showed that happiness spreads through social networks, affecting not only friends but friends of friends. "Our research showed that a person is 15 percent more likely to be happy if a close contact is happy as well," he explains.

Building Block: Sturdy Bones

A strong skeleton provides the foundation for an active lifestyle, essential for biking through wine country, tending your vegetables, and romping with your grandkids.

YOUR MOM'S MIDDLE AGE: She got plenty of calcium and vitamin D, both of which are crucial to maintaining bone mass.

THE NEW MIDDLE AGE: Add protein to the mix. "In addition to calcium and D, which are very important, you need a steady supply of protein to keep bones strong," explains Robert P. Heaney, MD, a professor of medicine at Creighton University Medical Center and a leading expert on osteoporosis. He believes dairy products such as milk and yogurt are the best sources of calcium because they contain the whole suite of nutrients, including protein, that you need for healthy bones. Boosting vitamin D with supplements (take at least 1,000 IU daily) is particularly important as you get older, he points out, because the skin becomes less efficient at generating this crucial nutrient from sunlight.

Building Block: Deft Balance

Skiing, tennis, biking, even ballroom dancing all require excellent balance, particularly the ability to recover quickly from an unexpected bump or slip.

One-third of older adults suffer tumbles, and serious falls can hamper your ability to remain active.

YOUR MOM'S MIDDLE AGE: She walked and did light aerobics, believing that just staying in reasonably good shape would suffice.

THE NEW MIDDLE AGE: Lift and flex. "Exercises that promote balance, flexibility, and strength are equally important," says Bonita Lynn Beattie, a physical therapist and vice president for injury prevention at the Center for Healthy Aging in Washington, DC. "Dance classes, tai chi, and yoga are all great activities for preserving a strong sense of balance." Also make sure you're getting adequate vitamin D. A study in the *Journal of the American Geriatrics Society* found that older people who took an 800 IU supplement daily had 72 percent fewer falls.

Building Block: Up-to-Date Vaccinations

Illnesses that can be prevented with vaccines cause almost 50,000 deaths a year in the United States and make many more people needlessly ill. Staying current is a proven lifesaver.

YOUR MOM'S MIDDLE AGE: She thought immunization was for kids. Her outdated view still persists, according to a 2007 survey by the National Foundation for Infectious Diseases. The organization found that 40 percent of American adults wrongly believe that because they got shots as a child, they don't need to worry about vaccinations.

THE NEW MIDDLE AGE: Get your shots. Only 42 percent of people ages 50 to 64 typically get yearly flu shots. Shingles, an excruciatingly painful disease caused by the varicella-zoster virus, strikes one in three Americans, yet only 2 percent of those age 60 and older have received the vaccine that can prevent the infection or reduce its painful symptoms. Tetanus-diphtheria boosters are recommended every 10 years, which is protection many people in middle age neglect. The next time you see your doctor, ask if you're due for any shots.

CHAPTER 4

Do-It-Yourself DNA TESTING

At-home genetic tests are all the rage. But can they really calculate your risk of developing life-threatening diseases? Before buying one, read this Prevention *special report.*

Anna Peterson is only 27, but she's already watched her mother and her aunt develop breast cancer. She also saw her grandmother's eyesight fail from macular degeneration. So Peterson, a graduate student in Ottawa, Ontario, took her health care into her own hands and did what millions of others of all ages are doing: She opted for an at-home genetic test.

When the results from the $985 test arrived in her e-mail, Peterson felt relief to learn that she didn't have an elevated genetic risk for macular degeneration. Yet the test did show a slightly elevated risk for the more common forms of breast cancer. The results, Peterson says, empowered her to make healthier choices. Together with her physician, she'll use that information to advocate for earlier screening for breast cancer and possibly start getting mammograms at age 30.

"Prevention starts with knowing the odds," says Peterson. "I now have the opportunity to make lifestyle changes in my 20s, rather than in my 60s."

Welcome to the brave new world of genetic testing. Once the exclusive domain of doctors and genetic counselors, DNA analysis is now a do-it-yourself proposition, with several dozen companies marketing tests directly to consumers, claiming that they will allow you to understand your genetic profile. The process is surprisingly simple: Buy a test online, swab the inside of your cheek or spit into a test tube to collect a DNA sample, and then mail it to the company. In return, you'll receive personalized medical information that purportedly helps you to combat disease by making informed choices about your health. Bolstering that promise is new research that shows you can actually turn off genes that promote certain diseases by improving your diet and managing better stress.

GENETIC TESTING GOES MAINSTREAM

People clearly approve of genetic testing. In a recent Prevention.com poll, 87 percent of respondents said they'd want to know which inherited diseases they're at high risk of developing. Moreover, 54 percent said they'd be likely to have a genetic test even if there was no known treatment or way to prevent the disease.

Plenty of companies are eager to meet this demand, selling at-home tests that range in cost from hundreds to thousands of dollars. Some offer tests that have long been available through doctors and genetic counselors—for instance, those that check for BRCA 1 or 2, the genes linked to a small percentage of inherited cases of breast cancer. Newer versions look at your SNPs (pronounced snips, short for "single nucleotide polymorphisms"), the slight variations within DNA that can account for differences in appearance and how we develop diseases.

The companies don't predict that you're going to get, say, cancer or macular degeneration. Rather, you get back a report showing the risk you run compared to the average person. One of the newest entrants into the at-home arena, Navigenics, recently launched its $2,500 Health Compass test, which looks for markers associated with 23 common conditions—including diabetes, prostate cancer, and Alzheimer's disease—that are "actionable," or able to be prevented or detected early. For an additional $250 per year, subscribers receive personalized updates when relevant genetic research—for instance, the discovery of new SNPs—changes their health outlook.

Health-conscious consumers are clearly enamored of these high-tech tests. They're expected to spend an estimated $6 billion to have their DNA decoded over the next 5 years. But while the business of do-it-yourself genetic testing is booming, experts say this new frontier of medicine isn't ready for prime time. They worry that the field is insufficiently regulated, not all of the tests are reliable, and the information garnered is incomplete and possibly misleading.

"Some tests lack adequate scientific evidence to support their use, and the lack of regulation means there's no way for consumers to separate the good from the bad," says Gail Javitt, JD, MPH, a research scholar at Johns Hopkins University.

THE RISKS OF PEERING INTO YOUR MEDICAL FUTURE

Despite an explosion in the discovery of SNPs, most experts say it's too early to make strong links between these tiny genetic variants and the development of diseases. That's because the role played by a single mutation is believed to be modest. Rather, it's the interaction between multiple SNPs and factors like diet, exercise, and weight that predispose you to disease. Indeed, studies show that lifestyle accounts for about 70 percent of our susceptibility to health problems such as diabetes, heart disease, and some types of cancer.

As a result, "these tests can't accurately predict the risk of developing these complex diseases at the moment," says David Hunter, ScD, MPH, a professor of epidemiology and nutrition at the Harvard School of Public Health. Likewise, some tests that claim to gauge your risk of diseases such as depression examine single genes that explain only a small part of the predisposition to those illnesses.

BREAKTHROUGH: SHOULD YOU CUSTOMIZE YOUR DRUGS TO YOUR DNA?

Here's a shocker: Due to differences in DNA, up to 60 percent of the most common drugs are associated with adverse reactions. This includes medication used to treat common conditions such as hypertension, heart failure, depression, high cholesterol, and asthma.

Hence the hope being pinned on pharmacogenetics, a field of medicine that promises to improve health care by allowing doctors to customize medical treatment to suit a person's unique genetic signature. Though experts predict that it could be decades before personalized medicine becomes the norm, research is moving ahead: Last fall, for instance, researchers at Duke University reported that people with a specific genetic variant saw less reduction in LDL, or "bad" cholesterol, when taking statins.

But for some drugs, the future is now. A genetic test recently approved by the FDA should help doctors determine the optimal dose of warfarin (Coumadin), a blood thinner used by 1 million Americans. Determining the right dose is crucial: Too much may result in an increased risk of excessive bleeding, while too little may cause a potentially fatal blood clot. By one estimate, using DNA analysis to

Critics also note that test results can be tough to interpret, making it difficult to know when and if you should take action. A Navigenics test told Robert C. Green, MD, MPH, a professor of neurology, genetics, and epidemiology at Boston University Schools of Medicine and Public Health, that he had a 20 percent above-average risk of developing multiple sclerosis. But the average risk is 0.3 percent, and his was just 0.5 percent. These are both very low risks (3 out of every 1,000 versus 5 out of every 1,000, respectively), yet the results were highlighted in orange, indicating an elevated risk. Green, a geneticist, understood his real risk, but the average person might not, causing needless worry.

And consider the flip side: that someone who tests negative for a gene or is

prescribe warfarin would prevent about 17,000 strokes and 85,000 serious bleeding incidents.

A small but growing number of doctors and hospitals are also using genetic testing to tailor treatment for the following medicines:

TAMOXIFEN: DNA testing identifies the 8 percent of women with genetic variants that keep them from metabolizing the breast cancer drug, rendering it ineffective.

PAINKILLERS SUCH AS CODEINE: Up to 8 percent of whites and 2 percent of Asians and African Americans are poor metabolizers of these drugs and won't get relief from them; for the 1 percent of "ultrarapid metabolizers," risks include respiratory problems.

ANTIDEPRESSANTS AND ANTIPSYCHOTICS: Some of these drugs are metabolized by the CYP2D6 and CYP2C19 genes. In 2005, the FDA approved a test that looks for these gene variations, and companies now sell consumer versions. But experts advise against using the at-home tests without having your doctor interpret the results, notes Julie Johnson, PharmD, professor of pharmacy and medicine at the University of Florida. The reason: These genes are involved in the metabolization of 25 percent of all prescription drugs, including several in which they play a very important role. If you misinterpret the results of an at-home test (and mistakenly think you don't have the gene), you might avoid taking one or more drugs you really need.

told she's at low risk for developing a dreaded disease becomes less motivated to lead a healthy lifestyle. David L. Katz, MD, MPH, director of the Prevention Research Center at Yale University School of Medicine, points to a study on premenopausal women given a range of tests to determine their risks of developing heart disease. Half saw scans of their coronary arteries, which were surprisingly healthy. But despite other risks revealed from triglyceride and blood glucose levels, the group that saw its healthy scans did less to follow recommendations to prevent heart disease.

"We don't want a single test talking people out of taking care of themselves, and this study suggests that can happen," says Dr. Katz.

TEST RESULTS: HELPFUL OR CONFUSING?

Proponents of mail-order genetic testing claim it has just the opposite effect and instead helps people gain new insights that sometimes dramatically boost their health. David Agus, MD, an oncologist and cancer researcher at the University of Southern California, started Navigenics with the hope that people would get tested, discuss results with their physicians, and use the information to seek earlier diagnoses or delay the onset or prevent certain conditions altogether. That's precisely what happened in the case of Mari Baker, the company's former CEO. When her results revealed a 5-times-greater risk of celiac disease, follow-up testing ordered by her physician confirmed she had the digestive disease, which is caused by an intolerance to gluten, a protein in wheat, rye, and barley. The diagnosis explained the gastrointestinal problems Baker, 45, suffered over the years. She immediately changed her diet and stocked her kitchen with gluten-free pasta, bread, and beer.

"Feeling a little bit better every day for the next 20 years is pretty important," she says.

Unfortunately, test results aren't always so clear-cut and accurate. Mike Spear, the communications director for a genomic research nonprofit in Alberta, took tests from deCODEme and 23andMe and received some conflicting findings. For instance, the deCODEme test showed a higher-than-average risk for MS, but the 23andMe test said his risk was no higher than that of the average person. The test from deCODEme also had a big check mark next to "male pattern baldness," while the 23andMe test said he was on par with the rest of the population. (Spear, who's 56, still has plenty of hair.) Most surprisingly, both tests told Spear that his risk of asthma was no different from the average person's, even though he already suffers from the disease. His impression: "I'd be careful about basing your life around genetic test results."

Although new genetic research emerges every day, scientists haven't discovered all the genetic variants—or all the SNPs—for common diseases. Shane Green, PhD, director of outreach at the Ontario Genomics Institute in Toronto, took two genetic tests, one from 23andMe and the other from Navigenics, and both told him that he had an average risk of cardiac disease. Yet he had undergone triple bypass heart surgery the previous year. As a runner who is not overweight, doesn't smoke, and has low cholesterol, Green suspects there's a genetic cause for his tendency toward blocked arteries. He chalks up the discrepancy in his test results to the fact that more research is needed to fully understand the genetic causes of cardiac disease.

Another reason to think twice about these tests: The industry is a virtual free-for-all. No single government agency watches the labs performing the tests to ensure that the science behind the tests is even real. Currently, the FDA reviews most other home-use medical tests for safety and effectiveness, but at-home genetic tests don't fall under the agency's aegis. Pending legislation would require makers of direct-to-consumer genetic tests to prove that their tests are accurate and properly performed.

But right now, "the public's best approach is buyer beware," says Kathy Hudson, PhD, founder and former director of the Genetics and Public Policy Center at Johns Hopkins.

Despite these warnings, experts predict that people will be very tempted by the chance to peek into the genetic crystal ball. If you're one of them, heed Dr. Katz's reminder: "DNA isn't destiny." And be aware that when it comes to the lifestyle choices that are the greatest predictors of health, your future is in your hands.

WHICH GENETIC TESTS MAKE THE GRADE?

Decent

TESTS FOR DISEASES WITH A PROVEN LINK TO SINGLE GENES. Unlike SNPs tests, which look at gene variations that may put you at higher risk for diseases, some tests screen for specific gene mutations that have been scientifically proven to either definitively cause a disease or greatly increase your chance of developing one. Some disorders that can be screened for this way include breast cancer, colon cancer, Huntington's (a neurological disorder), and hemochromatosis (when the body stores too much iron). When people concerned about these diseases want to protect their privacy, some opt to use at-home versions of tests so the results won't become part of medical records. Companies that offer this type of testing include DNA Direct, Kimball Genetics, and Myriad Genetics.

Consider with Caution

SNPS TESTS FROM COMPANIES THAT USE A LABORATORY CERTIFIED BY THE CLINICAL LABORATORY IMPROVEMENT AMENDMENTS. CLIA sets standards for US clinical laboratories, and accreditation ensures that the company uses laboratories that adhere to standards and guidelines for clinical testing. Companies using CLIA-certified labs include DNA Direct and Navigenics.

COMPANIES THAT OFFER GENETIC COUNSELING. Some genetic tests deal with statistical risk that can be tough to understand and needs to be considered with your family history, so be sure a knowledgeable health professional interprets your test to avoid needless anxiety and rash medical decisions. Some companies include free online or telephone sessions with certified genetic counselors and send detailed reports to help explain what test results really mean.

Avoid

"NUTRIGENOMIC" TESTS. These promise to identify your risk of certain diseases and then sell you expensive vitamin regimes that are supposedly based on your genetic profile and help you prevent disease. The General Accounting Office (GAO), the investigative arm of Congress, looked at a number of these companies and found that some of these recommended supplements cost $1,200 a year and were actually similar to supplements found in stores for $35. In some cases, the vitamins exceeded recommended daily allowances, making them potentially harmful, and regardless of different DNA samples, the "personalized" supplements sent to customers were all the same. GAO investigators couldn't verify any of the scientific claims made by manufacturers of these tests.

TESTS FROM COMPANIES WITHOUT STRICT PRIVACY POLICIES. Despite passage in 2008 of the Genetic Information Nondiscrimination Act, which prohibits your insurance company and employer from using your genetic information against you, no laws yet exist to limit what genetic testing companies can and cannot do with a person's genetic information or DNA sample. Be sure that a company securely stores your DNA sample and will not sell it to be used in a research study without your permission. If the company doesn't provide this information on its Web site, ask for it directly. "Using your information without your consent is unethical," says Caroline Lieber, MS, director of the graduate program in human genetics at Sarah Lawrence College.

TESTS THAT DON'T PROVIDE DOCUMENTED SCIENTIFIC EVIDENCE VALIDATING THEIR CLAIMS. You should be fully informed about what a test can and cannot say about your health. Companies should make scientific references available on their Web sites to document the data used for the tests. If they don't offer it, ask for it.

CHAPTER 5

Top To-Do's for
WELLNESS

Simple ways to leave your Lysol and
stay germ-free

Your body is capable of many amazing things, but perhaps none is as extraordinary as its ability to protect you from infection. Millions of cells, each with a highly specialized function, communicate and collaborate with each other not only to destroy pathogens but also to remember them should they try to invade again.

All this goes on without your even realizing it—well, except for the occasional microbe that slips through undetected. Given the sheer volume of germs that you encounter on a daily basis, your immune system's track record is quite impressive.

But it needs proper care and feeding to keep on doing what it does so well. That's where you come in. By taking steps to strengthen your immune function and reduce your germ exposure, you can greatly improve your odds of not getting sick.

We're not asking you to reinvent your lifestyle for the sake of staying healthy, because you really don't need to. As you'll see in this chapter, sometimes the simplest changes can yield the most dramatic results.

With guidance from our team of health experts, we've put together the following list of best practices to keep your immune system primed for action and to knock germs off their game. These tips are effective, easy to use, and even a bit unexpected.

EAT FOR GOOD HEALTH, NOT JUST IMMUNITY

Why it works: A healthy diet nourishes your entire body, not just certain parts, explains David L. Katz, MD, MPH, director of the Prevention Research Center at Yale University School of Medicine. "You need white blood cells for good immunity, and they require good bone marrow to form and a healthy heart and blood vessels to travel throughout your body," he says. "All of your body's systems are interrelated. That's why robust immunity equals robust health—and why healthy eating is really a holistic thing."

Where to start: Your body will thrive on a diet that features whole grains, fruits and vegetables, and lean proteins such as chicken and fish. Nuts, seeds, olive oil, and avocados are good choices for monounsaturated fats. And don't forget fatty fish like salmon and mackerel for a healthy dose of omega-3 fatty acids.

What your body doesn't need are refined grains, sugars, and the saturated fats in red meats and full-fat dairy products. Try to limit these as much as possible.

→ PREVENTION
Alert!

FOOD'S COLD-COMFORT ZONE

Keep a basic thermometer in your refrigerator and make sure it doesn't rise above 40°F, suggest Tennessee State University researchers. Cold stifles bacterial growth, preventing spoilage. Yet only 10 percent of fridge owners keep a thermometer inside (the "coldness dial" doesn't cut it). Install one, check it daily, and store perishables such as dairy on the top shelf (the coldest area) and away from the fridge door. Nearly 40 percent of doors topped 40°F for 24 hours straight, even when left closed.

For extra credit: Here's a super-easy strategy to make sure that you're getting the proper mix of foods and nutrients at every meal. Imagine that your dinner plate is divided into quarters. Two of those quarters should be occupied by veggies and fruits. One-quarter should have whole grains, and the remaining one-quarter lean protein.

PICK BRIGHTLY COLORED PRODUCE

Why it works: Pretty much any fruit or veggie has something to offer your immune system. But for immune-boosting prowess, says Ann Kulze, MD, founder and CEO of Just Wellness LLC and author of *Dr. Ann's 10-Step Diet*, these are the cream of the crop: berries, whole citrus fruits, kiwi, apples, red grapes, kale, onions, spinach, sweet potatoes, and carrots. What do they have in common? Their eye-catching colors, which tell you at a glance that they're loaded with phytochemicals.

"The interesting thing about phytochemicals is that when they're isolated in supplement form, they seem to lose their immune-boosting benefits," Dr. Kulze notes. "That's why eating fruits and vegetables is the best strategy for getting the hundreds of micronutrients that work synergistically to enhance your immunity."

Where to start: Choose fresh fruits and veggies when in season, frozen at other times of year. How you eat them is up to you! For example, you might sprinkle berries on your morning cereal, toss spinach and kale into a salad, or nibble on baby carrots for an afternoon snack. The possibilities are endless!

For extra credit: Pair your produce with other healthy foods for a more powerful immune punch. You might mix your berries into yogurt containing active cultures, the beneficial bacteria that help keep the bad bugs in check. Or serve up a sweet potato as a side dish to wild salmon, which is rich in omega-3 fatty acids.

BE UNCONVENTIONAL—GO ORGANIC!

Why it works: To most of us, a vegetable is a vegetable and a fruit is a fruit. But some of our experts, including Neal Barnard, MD, president of the

Physicians Committee for Responsible Medicine in Washington, DC, believe that organic is the only choice if your goal is to ensure the robust function of your immune system.

One reason is that organic produce is more nutritious, with improved vitamin and mineral content, according to studies. Two, it contains fewer pesticides, among other chemicals.

The jury is out on just how harmful pesticides are, but in Dr. Barnard's opinion, "It's likely choosing organic products will result in lower cancer rates and, for women who are pregnant, fewer birth defects."

Where to start: If you're still on the fence about organics, you needn't be a complete convert. Instead, try making the switch for just those fruits and veggies with the greatest pesticide content. As a general rule, peaches, apples, and bell peppers rank high for contaminants, while onions, avocados, and frozen sweet corn are largely contaminant-free. For a list of foods and their pesticide scores, visit www.foodnews.org.

For extra credit: Before buying organic produce at the supermarket, check out what's available at your local farmers' market. "I am quite certain that I can find organic produce grown under large-scale farming conditions that is potentially less nutritious than produce grown locally," says Christopher Gardner, PhD, an associate professor in the Prevention Research Center at Stanford School of Medicine.

MAKE OMEGA-3s YOUR FAVORITE FAT

Why it works: Omega-3s help reduce inflammation, which is a factor in colds and flu, among many other conditions. If the latest research is any indication, that may be just one aspect of how these beneficial fats contribute to immunity.

"Omega-3s are almost like the CEOs at the cellular level," Dr. Kulze says. "They create building blocks within the cells that drive the body's immune response."

Where to start: Currently, there are no official guidelines for omega-3 intake. To get the most from these beneficial fats, the American Heart

MICROWAVE DOS AND DONT'S

More than 90 percent of US homes have a microwave. Although immeasurably convenient, they're not foolproof when it comes to food safety. Here's how to use yours without harm:

DO: Cook leftovers until they're steaming hot. They can still harbor dangerous bacteria if not warmed to 165°F throughout. If there are cold spots, stir, rotate, and reheat.

DON'T: Ignore instructions calling for standing or resting time. Microwaves cook from the outside in, usually to a depth of only 1 to 1½ inches. When a food rests, it's using conduction to heat more thoroughly.

DO: Use microwave-safe cookware. Avoid dishes or containers that are metallic, including decorative paint and trim, which can cause sparks to form when heated. And skip plastic take-out bowls and food containers, as well as plastic wraps and foam trays, such as those used for ground beef and turkey: They may leach harmful chemicals into foods when heated.

Association recommends eating a serving of fish—particularly fatty fish like mackerel, lake trout, herring, sardines, albacore tuna, and salmon—at least twice a week.

For extra credit: Although food should be your primary source of any nutrient, including omega-3s, Dr. Katz says this is one instance where supplementing may make good sense. "The typical American diet contains too many omega-6 fatty acids and not enough omega-3s," he notes. "A supplement can help restore proper balance."

Dr. Kulze likes a product called Nordic Naturals Omega-3D, which combines fish oil with another immune booster, vitamin D. To learn more about this product, visit www.nordicnaturals.com.

USE GARLIC LIBERALLY

Why it works: Vampires aren't the only ones to be repelled by garlic. Bacteria and viruses are averse to its properties, too. The pungent bulb is an established germ fighter, and it enhances immunity.

Garlic owes its therapeutic properties to allicin, which is the chemical compound that's responsible for its very distinctive smell. Allicin increases both natural killer cells and T-lymphocytes, the white blood cells that seek out and destroy invading pathogens.

"It's believed that people who ate a lot of raw garlic were the ones who survived the plague," says Susan Schenck, coauthor of *The Live Food Factor*.

WIPE OUT THE 10 WORST GERM HOT SPOTS

You might scrub your toilet and countertops until they shine, but when it comes to the war between you and germs, consider yourself outnumbered. Germs (the catchall name for bacteria, viruses, and other microorganisms) are everywhere—at home, in the office, even in your car. Luckily, about 99 percent of them can't harm us. But the other 1 percent can be annoying, uncomfortable, or downright scary: Most of these pathogens are either viral or bacterial and can cause everything from a runny nose to a potentially life-threatening infection.

You might think you know the obvious places that germs propagate—the doctor's office, the soles of your shoes—but many more germ-friendly locales are completely unexpected yet no less dangerous. We uncovered a host of surprising new spots where germs like to lurk, and we offer easy solutions to keep you and your family safe and healthy.

THE KITCHEN FAUCET. That metal aeration screen at the end of your kitchen faucet reduces water flow, which is good for the environment, but not so much for your health: Running water keeps the screen moist, an ideal condition for bacteria growth. Because tap water is far from sterile, if you accidentally touch the screen with dirty fingers or food, bacteria can grow on the faucet, explains microbiologist Kelly Reynolds, PhD, an associate professor of community environment and policy at the University of Arizona Zuckerman College of Public Health. Over time, bacteria build up and form a wall of

Where to start: To get the most benefit from garlic, use the fresh stuff. "Fresh garlic that you mince yourself is a lot more potent than the dried or processed kind that you find at the supermarket," Dr. Kulze says. She recommends cutting it up about 10 to 15 minutes before you plan to use it.

For extra credit: Eating raw garlic isn't for the fainthearted; many people find the smell and taste overpowering. But cooking garlic can reduce its antimicrobial effects. If possible, try not to add it until the very end of the cooking process to help preserve its allicin content. Then stir it into soups and sauces, sprinkle it over fajitas and stir-fries, and use it as a garnish on steaks and burgers. Just remember, a little garlic goes a long way!

---

pathogens called biofilm that sticks to the screen. "Eventually, that biofilm may even be big enough to break off and get onto your food or dishes," she notes.

Keep it clean: Once a week, remove the screen and soak it in a diluted bleach solution (follow the directions on the label). Replace the screen, and let the water run a few minutes before using.

THE GARBAGE DISPOSAL. That raw chicken or spinach you re rinsing for dinner is often loaded with harmful bacteria, which can make the young, the elderly, or anyone with a compromised immune system seriously ill. In fact, there are often more than 500,000 bacteria in the kitchen sink—about 1,000 times more than the average toilet has. Although the metal part of the disposal produces ions that can help kill germs, they still love to grow on the crevices in and around the slimy rubber stopper. That means your disposal can become party central for bacteria, contaminating whatever touches it—dishes, utensils, even your hands.

Keep it clean: At least once a week, clean the disposal's rubber stopper with a diluted bleach solution; soap and water aren't enough.

THE WELCOME MAT. It serves to greet not only your guests but also all the bugs on the bottoms of their shoes. One study found that nearly 96 percent of shoe soles had traces of *coliform,* which includes fecal bacteria. "The area near your front door is one of the dirtiest in the house," says Dr. Reynolds. Once bacteria put down stakes in your mat, anytime you walk on it you give them a free ride into your home.

(continued)

Keep it clean: Spray the doormat once a week with a fabric-safe disinfectant (such as Lysol Disinfectant Spray). Leave shoes at the door, and avoid resting bags and groceries on the mat, too.

YOUR VACUUM CLEANER. "Vacuums—including the brushes and bags—are like meals-on-wheels for bacteria," says Charles P. Gerba, PhD, professor and environmental microbiologist at the University of Arizona. "You suck in all this bacteria and food, creating an atmosphere for growth." A recent study by Dr. Gerba and his team found that 13 percent of all vacuum cleaner brushes tested positive for *E. coli,* which means you could spread it around the house each time you use the appliance.

Keep it clean: Change your vacuum bag frequently, and do so outdoors to avoid the cloud of bacteria that filters into the air. (Vacuum bags that feature antibacterial linings are best, and they are available for many major brands.) Clean the cavity of a bagless vacuum with diluted bleach and let it air-dry.

A DISH TOWEL. You know a sponge can harbor nasty germs, but a recent study of hundreds of homes across the United States found that about 7 percent of kitchen towels were contaminated with MRSA (methicillin-resistant *Staphylococcus aureus),* the difficult-to-treat staph bacteria that can cause life-threatening skin infections. Dish towels also rated tops for dangerous strains of *E. coli* and other bacteria. We often use towels to wipe up spills, says Dr. Reynolds, and then reuse them before washing them, which spreads germs.

Keep it clean: Stick to paper towels to clean countertops, and save the dish towel to dry just-washed pots and plates. Change towels or launder at least twice a week in hot water and bleach.

YOUR CAR'S DASHBOARD. In tests of 100 vehicles from across the United States, the dashboard was found to be the second-most-common spot for bacteria and mold. (Food spills were number one.) The researchers' rationale: When air—which carries mold spores and bacteria—gets sucked in through the vents, it's often drawn to the dashboard, where it can deposit the spores and germs. Because the dashboard receives the most sun and tends to stay warm, it's prime for growth.

Keep it clean: Regularly swipe the inside of your car with disinfecting wipes. Be more vigilant during allergy season. About 20 million Americans are affected by asthma, which is caused in part by an allergic reaction to mold.

SOAP DISPENSERS. Soap that harbors bacteria may sound ironic, but one recent study found that about 25 percent of liquid soap dispensers in public restrooms were contaminated by fecal bacteria. "Most of these containers are never cleaned, so bacteria grows as the soap scum builds up," says Dr. Gerba. "And the bottoms are touched by dirty hands, so there's a continuous culture going on feeding millions of bacteria."

Keep it clean: Be sure to scrub hands thoroughly for 15 to 20 seconds with plenty of hot water, and if you have an alcohol gel disinfectant, use that, too.

RESTAURANT KETCHUP BOTTLE. It's the rare eatery that regularly bleaches condiment containers. And the reality is that many people don't wash their hands before eating, says Dr. Reynolds. So while you may be diligent, the guy who poured the ketchup before you may not have been, which means his germs are now on your fries.

Keep it clean: Squirt hand sanitizer on the outside of the bottle or use a disinfectant wipe before you grab it. Holding the bottle with a napkin won't help. They're porous, so microorganisms can walk right through, says Dr. Reynolds.

THE REFRIGERATOR SEAL. A University of Arizona survey of 160 homes in three US cities found that the seal around the fridge tested positive 83 percent of the time for common molds. The mold can spread every time the refrigerator door opens—exposing anyone who's susceptible to allergies and potentially contaminating the food.

Keep it clean: Wipe fridge seals at least once a week with a diluted bleach solution or disinfectant.

YOUR CELL PHONE. You probably put it down anyplace that's convenient, but consider this: Several studies on cell phones and PDAs found that they carry tons of bacteria, including *Staph* (which can cause skin infections), *Pseudomonas* (eye infections), and *Salmonella* (stomach ailments). Many electronic devices are sheathed in leather or vinyl cases, which provide plenty of creases and crevices for germs to hide.

Keep it clean: Use a disinfecting wipe a few times a week, and be conscious of where you rest personal items.

CHAPTER 6

ALLERGY
Breakthroughs

Surprising places where irritants lurk, and easy ways to get rid of them

Seasonal allergies are the bane of the approximately 35 million Americans. Pollen may not be all that's making your eyes water and nose run, though. Surprising allergens lurk in unexpected places in your home and make you feel even worse. In fact, the list of sneeze-inducing culprits is long: animal dander, mold, dust, and dust mites (tiny insects that thrive on organic matter, primarily flakes of skin) as well as pollen carried into the house from outside. But these irritants are manageable, and getting a handle on them will help reduce your symptoms. We went to four top experts for the unexpected sources of your sneezes and some room-by-room tips for eliminating them.

LIVING ROOM

Surprise allergy source: Pet-owning visitors. Friends with pets usually have animal dander on their clothes. When they visit, they can deposit this irritant on upholstered furniture—even if they don't bring Fido or Felix with them.

Solution: Vacuum your couches and padded chairs after pet-owning pals sit on them. Prevent the allergens from spewing right back out of the machine by using one with a HEPA filter, which traps tiny particles so they can't escape the dust bag.

Surprise allergy sources: Couch pillows, throws, and stuffed toys. These items come into contact with skin, and that means tiny flakes that slough off and encourage dust mites. If your pet sits on, fetches, or plays with any of these, they're also covered with animal dander.

Solution: Tumble the items in the dryer on high for 10 to 15 minutes each week. (If this will damage the material, clean instead according to the manufacturer's instructions.)

BEDROOM

Surprise allergy source: Shelves. It's not just your novel's plot twists that are causing your eyes to tear up and your nose to run. You can also blame the

---

OUR EXPERTS

The following authorities supplied the information in this chapter.

Jeff May, certified indoor air quality professional, former board member of the Asthma and Allergy Foundation of America, coauthor of *Jeff May's Healthy Home Tips*

Morris Nejat, MD, New York Allergy & Sinus Centers

James Seltzer, MD, chairman of the Indoor Allergy Committee of the American College of Allergy, Asthma & Immunology

James Sublett, MD, managing partner, Family Allergy and Asthma, Louisville, Kentucky

dust that collects on books and other shelf-dwellers, including framed photographs and mementos. Books can also contribute to indoor mold problems, especially in humid conditions.

Solution: Keep shelves of all kinds, including bookshelves, away from the bed, or banish them from the bedroom entirely. Place trinkets behind glass doors so they don't collect dust. Clean surfaces and vacuum bedroom floors at least once a week.

Surprise allergy source: Bed pillows. The warmth and humidity of your body encourage dust mites to grow in bed pillows, no matter what type of stuffing they have.

Solution: Either trade old pillows for new ones annually, or encase pillows in allergy-proof covers that you wash once or twice a month in hot water (follow the manufacturer's instructions). The most allergy-resistant, comfortable cases are made of tightly woven fabric that's impermeable to dust mites and feels good to the touch. Check out the options at www.allergybuyersclub.com and www.nationalallergy.com.

BATHROOM

Surprise allergy source: The floor mat. Trapped moisture in the bath mat causes dust mites and mold to thrive.

Solution: Choose a washable mat and clean it weekly. (But never put a rubber-backed mat into the dryer.) After a shower or steamy bath, hang it up and open a window or run the fan.

KITCHEN

Surprise allergy source: The refrigerator door seal. As you transfer food in and out of the refrigerator, moisture, crumbs, and spills can build up in the crevices of the door seal and encourage mold to flourish there.

Solution: Wipe the seal with a mixture of mold-zapping bleach and water weekly; use a cotton swab to get into the grooves and clean them thoroughly.

Surprise allergy source: Cooking steam. Steam wafts from pots and pans as you cook and settles in places you may not clean daily, causing mold to build up. Spots where dampness may land include walls, ceilings, cupboard doors, upper shelves, and areas hidden behind large appliances.

Solution: Run the stove's exhaust fan to vent cooking moisture, not just smells, out of the house. If mold does appear, eliminate it with a solution of bleach and water.

LAUNDRY ROOM

Surprise allergy source: Damp clothes. Mold and bacteria can develop on damp, unwashed clothing that sits around for days before it's laundered, as well as on clean items left in the washer tub for more than a few hours.

62 THE PERCENTAGE OF PEOPLE WHO SUFFER FROM ALLERGIES WHO SAY THAT THEIR SYMPTOMS AFFECT THEIR MOODS

STOP SNEEZIN'

The following things can actually make your allergies worse.

Stressful Deadlines

In a 2008 experiment, researchers at Ohio State University College of Medicine found that allergy sufferers had more symptoms after they took an anxiety-inducing test, compared with when they performed a task that did not make them tense. Stress hormones may stimulate the production of IgE, blood proteins that cause allergic reactions, says study author Janice Kiecolt-Glaser, PhD.

GET RELIEF: If you're under stress, get enough sleep. A sleep deficit can worsen both allergy symptoms and stress, she says.

An Extra Glass of Wine

Alcohol can raise the risk of perennial allergic rhinitis by 3 percent for every additional alcoholic beverage consumed each week, Danish researchers found. One potential reason: Bacteria and yeast in the alcohol produce histamines, chemicals that cause telltale allergy symptoms like stuffy nose and itchy eyes.

GET RELIEF: Avoid alcohol when your symptoms are acting up, says Richard F. Lockey, MD, director of the Division of Allergy and Immunology at the University of South Florida College of Medicine.

Waiting Too Long to Take Meds

Medications that block histamines work best before you're even exposed to allergens, says allergist James Sublett, MD, a spokesperson for the American College of Allergy, Asthma, and Immunology.

GET RELIEF: Start medication a couple of weeks before the season commences or before you'll be around allergens (if you react to grass, before a golf game, for example).

Solution: Don't let moist, dirty laundry build up, and dry freshly washed items ASAP. Here's a bonus idea: Use liquid detergent instead of powder, which can produce irritating dust, worsening your allergy symptoms.

ALL AROUND THE HOUSE

Surprise allergy sources: Your hair and clothes. When you arrive home after spending time outdoors, you carry in dust and pollen on your shoes and clothes and in your hair. Long hair and loose hairstyles tend to trap more irritants than short or tightly bound strands.

Solution: When outside, cover your hair with a hat or scarf. When you get home, remove your head covering and shoes inside the door, change into clothes that you wear only indoors, and shampoo and dry your hair. Wash your comb and brush weekly to keep them free of any irritants they've picked up.

Surprise allergy source: Plants. Damp soil can support the development of mold, and if you spill occasionally as you water, you can encourage growths in any carpet or curtains you happen to hit.

Solution: Give away or toss out plants if mold and dust cause you to have severe symptoms. If you choose to keep the plants, place the pots on tile and well away from curtains. Bonus tip: A layer of pebbles or small stones placed on top of the soil will prevent the release of mold spores that may be growing in the soil.

Surprise allergy source: The fish tank. Mold grows on parts of the tank or bowl that are out of the water but nevertheless remain damp. Carelessly strewn fish food also helps mold develop and can nourish a dust mite colony.

Solution: Use a rag to dry off above-water tank parts daily. When you feed the fish, make sure the food lands in the water, not on the tabletop or floor.

CONFESSIONS OF A HEALTH SNOB

I prided myself on chronic good health, until I realized you don't need a cold to deserve a little care.

by Joyce Maynard

"Don't hug me," says a friend, in a scene that plays out at least a dozen times every cold season. "I don't want you to catch what I've got."

"Cough on me all you like," I tell her. "I don't get sick."

That's not to brag; it's just a statement of fact. I virtually never set foot in a doctor's office, much less the hospital. My babies (three of them) were born at home, without complications. I'm like my mother—the healthiest woman I ever knew, until the day she died.

I am lucky for a lot of reasons, but the physical resilience I've enjoyed throughout my life is one of the most obvious. I wake up feeling good nearly every morning. On those rare occasions when I feel less than my best, I tend to keep that information concealed, sometimes even from myself.

Perhaps because of this, I have a hard time empathizing properly with other people's aches and pains. If a friend has her heart broken, I'll offer support. But when one of my sons got hemorrhoids on the day of a big bike ride, I wanted him to buck up and hop in the saddle. When a then-boyfriend expressed justifiable concern about getting malaria on a rugged trip we were planning into the Costa Rican jungle, I left him home.

Lately, I've been keeping company with a man who goes to doctors, takes medicine, and gets MRIs. A man who takes good care of me, too, I would add, and urges me to get checkups. "I'll even pay for it," he says, when I mention it's a waste of money for a person like me. Still, I get judgmental. Once, when I was irritated with his speculation concerning some new illness he thought he might have, I told him he had too much time on his hands. I was too busy to get sick, was my slightly sanctimonious message. Some of us have more important things to do with our lives.

It's an unattractive trait, this lack of sympathy, though it has recently occurred to me that the weakness I've denied most resolutely is my own. I never complain when I walk 50 blocks in uncomfortable shoes. When I gave birth, not only was it in my own bed, I hopped up afterward to change the sheets. I was too tough to ask for help.

And when I consider why this might be, I go back, once again, to my mother, who never got sick either. And to my father, who got sick a lot.

My father had only to read about an ailment to imagine he might have it. When I was little and my mother read me the story of the princess and the pea, I remember thinking that my father was precisely the type of person who would have suffered a sleepless night atop 20 mattresses if a pea was hidden under the bottom one. I wanted to be like my mother, who could have gotten a good night's sleep in a bathtub.

But when my mother was 66 and seemingly in the bloom of health, she collapsed on a sidewalk and was diagnosed with cancer. A few months later she died, leaving my sister and me reeling.

The words "I take after my mother" acquired a different meaning for me in the years since her death. She believed she couldn't get sick because nobody but her would be able to take care of things. There was some truth to that: She was married to an alcoholic, a deeply lovable man who needed caretaking. As for me, I've been a single parent for close to 2 decades. Like my mother, I had to keep marching no matter what—or at least that's what I believed.

"I can't afford to get sick," I used to say when my kids were young, not understanding, perhaps, that sometimes allowing one's self to get sick—or just to slow down, to rest—is something a person can't afford not to do.

My mother had a saying: "If I ever come down with a brain tumor"—then she would mention something she'd do for herself, like buy a dress at regular price or lie in a hammock all day and read. And then she got a brain tumor and didn't have time to do any of it. I was 35 years old then. I'm now 55. And what I know now is that a person shouldn't have to get a terminal diagnosis to justify a little self-indulgence. Or, simply, self-care.

I was in a minor car accident recently with my boyfriend. Nobody was seriously hurt, but he was badly thrown around, and so when the ambulance arrived, he asked to be put in one of those collars that stabilize the neck. As they were buckling it around him, he looked at me remorsefully. "I know you think I'm a baby," he said. "I'm sorry."

Maybe that's when it hit me, how far overboard I'd gone—that a good man, a loving man, who had just narrowly escaped serious injury, would actually be afraid I'd think less of him for not jogging away from the wreckage.

I spurned the neck brace that was offered to me. It was 2 days later that I realized I needed one and—for the first time in my life—called the chiropractor.

I needed something more, however: humility. A little late in the game, I am at last acquiring some. Never having aches and pains is not a virtue, I know now. And having them now and then is not a moral failing. So after I left the chiropractor, I called my boyfriend.

I'm not Superwoman after all, I told him. I actually feel lousy. He did not gloat. He offered sympathy. Everyone feels bad sometimes, he said. And you should take it easy when you do.

Part 2

WEIGHT-LOSS
WISDOM

CHAPTER 7

Little-Known Diet
SABOTEURS

Here's why some weight-loss strategies backfire, and the fixes that help you reach your goal.

If you're trying to slim down, you've probably amassed a menu full of calorie-cutting tips and tricks. So it may come as a shock to learn that many of the ones you've sworn by are actually keeping you fat.

"In their quest to lose weight, many women unknowingly sabotage themselves," says Elisa Zied, RD, an American Dietetic Association spokesperson and author of *Feed Your Family Right!*

Looking for some motivation? The benefits of weight loss are many. Here are just a few of our favorite quality-of-life rewards.

Fewer headaches. Obese adults had up to a 40 percent higher likelihood of severe headaches or migraines than did healthy-weight people in a recent Centers for Disease Control study.

Improved oral health. As many as 52 percent of overweight and obese adults have gum disease, compared with 14 percent of normal-weight adults, reports a recent study in the *Journal of Clinical Periodontology*.

Longer and deeper sleep. Overweight adults sleep less and wake more than normal-weight counterparts, say researchers at Penn State.

Brighter outlook. Overweight and obese women were up to 31 percent more likely to have depression than normal-weight women, according to a recent *International Journal of Obesity* study of more than 177,000 adults.

Here are six well-intentioned approaches to weight loss that can go awry and the expert and research-proven ways to drop pounds for good.

YOU SAVE YOUR CALORIES FOR A BIG DINNER

Yes, cutting total calories leads to weight loss. But bank most of those calories for the end of the day and your hunger hormones will go haywire, making you eat more. Middle-age men and women who ate their daily number of calories in one supersize supper produced more ghrelin, a hormone that causes hunger, than when they ate the same number of calories in three square meals, found researchers at the National Institute on Aging.

Smarter move: Front-load your calories. Overeating at night keeps you from being hungry in the morning, setting off a vicious cycle in which you're

PREVENTION Alert!

WHY YOUR SCALE MIGHT BE STUCK

Maybe you're cutting the wrong calories! Reducing "liquid calories" from beverages such as soda, fruit punch, and sweetened iced tea is 5 times more effective for weight loss than cutting back on calories from solid foods, finds a study in the *American Journal of Clinical Nutrition*. The researchers say that because swallowing beverages does not satiate the body the way chewing solid food does, it causes people to overeat.

never interested in breakfast but always starving by dinner. The key is to rebalance your day so you don't set yourself up for an evening binge.

To get your appetite back in the morning, cut your evening meal in half. Then eat a breakfast of about 450 calories, such as a scrambled egg with low-fat cheese on a whole wheat English muffin with an 8-ounce glass of juice, which is an amount that should keep you satisfied until lunch, says George L. Blackburn, MD, PhD, associate director of the division of nutrition at Harvard Medical School and author of *Break Through Your Set Point*. Once your appetite adjusts, don't go more than 5 hours without another meal of roughly the same size.

YOU GRAZE INSTEAD OF EATING REGULARLY SCHEDULED MEALS

Trouble is, eating in this manner may contribute to weight gain, according to a 2005 *American Journal of Clinical Nutrition* study. When researchers asked women to eat at regular, fixed times or to break their usual amount of food into unscheduled meals throughout the day, they made a startling discovery: The women actually burned more calories in the 3 hours after eating the regular meals than they did after the unplanned meals. They produced less insulin, too, potentially lowering their odds of insulin resistance, which is linked to weight gain and obesity.

What's more, grazing instead of planning ahead can set you up to eat mindlessly, says Zied. In the end, we rarely realize how many calories all those little nibbles and noshes really add up to.

Smarter move: Figure out how many times a day you need to eat—everybody is different—and then stick to a schedule.

"It's not great to feel starved, but it is okay to feel slightly hungry," says Zied. You can home in on your body's internal cues with a food diary. It's so effective that earlier this year, researchers at Kaiser Permanente Center for Health Research found that dieters who kept a food journal lost twice as much weight as those who didn't record what they ate.

MY "PERFECT" DIET IS MAKING ME FAT!

More vegetables, less red meat, no chips or soda. So if we're doing everything right, why is the needle on the scale going in the wrong direction? We asked two diet experts, Dawn Jackson Blatner, RD, author of *The Flexitarian Diet,* and New York City-based nutritionist Katherine Brooking, RD, to review the weeklong food diaries of people like us and find out. Even with the best of intentions, something as simple as a healthy-but-oversize snack can make us gain. But finding small ways to save just 100 calories a day can take off 10 pounds in a year. Learn from these women's mistakes. Their diet tweaks can help you reach your weight loss goals.

The Yo-Yo Dieter

"I eat healthy, balanced meals and snacks, and my weight still fluctuates."
—Belinda R., 54

For the past 25 years, Belinda has watched the numbers on the scale bounce up and down. Most recently, she shed 20 pounds before putting it right back on.

"I weigh 244 now, and I don't know why because overall, I think I eat well," she says. For Belinda, that means making sure each meal includes a healthy combination of fat, carbohydrates, and protein plus at least one fruit or vegetable—such as chicken and hummus in a multigrain wrap, with baby carrots on the side. For snacks and sometimes on-the-go meals, she'll rely on protein bars and shakes. Her one soft spot is cookies.

"I try to satisfy my cravings with lower-fat versions or mini cookies," she says. And to keep her "furnace stoked," Belinda eats every 3 hours, even setting her cell phone's alarm to remind her. She also drinks about 50 ounces of water a day, skips alcohol and fast food, and exercises regularly.

EXPERT FIX: "Eating every few hours is a good way to keep metabolism moving, but Belinda is consuming way too many calories," says Brooking. Her snacks are the culprits.

"They're too big and too frequent," explains Blatner. "Even though her choices are healthy, she's eating, on average, 800 calories in snacks, so it's like she's having two extra meals." Instead, she can stay satisfied eating just two snacks a day, at about 150 calories each. That alone would help her drop about a pound a week! Belinda should also go back to keeping a food diary, suggests Brooking. "It's helped her lose before because it keeps her accountable." Here are some more calorie-cutting tips.

PARE DOWN THE ENERGY BARS. Belinda will have a 400-calorie bar as a snack, when really, that's a meal, says Blatner. "She can have one protein bar or shake a day. Under 200 calories is a snack; anything higher counts as a meal."

GO LEAN ON PROTEIN. Although Brenda eats chicken, she often indulges in higher-fat proteins, particularly carne asada (thin slices of grilled beef) and tri tip, a triangular cut from the bottom of a sirloin. On some days, she'll have two servings of beef; on average, five a week. Belinda does weigh out the proper serving, but just 3 ounces of tri tip contains 225 calories, nearly half of which come from fat. The same amount of skinless turkey has 144 calories. And turkey sausage has 75 percent less saturated fat than the pork version. Other lean sources of protein are fish and beans.

SKIP "DIET" TREATS. Fat-free and sugar-free aren't necessarily low-calorie: For example, one brand of chocolate chip cookie has 53 calories; the reduced-fat version has only 6 fewer. Plus, studies show that overweight people who eat low-fat instead of regular snacks consume, on average, twice as many calories. To satisfy her cookie craving, Belinda should have about 150 calories' worth of the real thing, says Brooking.

The Food Cop

"I stick to small servings but can't lose the last 10 pounds." —Donna Gold, 56

Donna certainly doesn't eat a lot. She'll have a fat-free milk cappuccino for breakfast. "Food too early in the morning turns on my hunger switch, and then I'm looking for snacks all day," she explains. For lunch, she'll have a small yogurt-and-fruit shake, and dinner is often two pieces of chicken, spinach with walnuts as a side, and wine or beer. "Most nights, I don't eat until 9:30, so sometimes I'll skip a real meal and have handfuls of nuts and prunes," she says. Red meat is a rarity; so are rice and bread. Occasionally, she'll indulge in a few chocolates in the afternoon or a handful of chocolate chips after dinner. She does Pilates, rides a stationary bike, and tries to hike or ski on weekends. She carries 155 pounds on her 5-foot-4 frame and wants to drop 10 more. "It's so confusing," she says. "How can I eat so little and still not lose?"

(continued)

EXPERT FIX: Donna's right—on some days, it doesn't seem like she's eating enough to gain weight, and that might be part of her problem, says Brooking: "If she gets less than 1,200 calories in a day, her metabolism will slow down to help conserve energy and prevent starvation." To reach her goal, she should consume about 1,450 calories a day and spread out her meals and snacks more evenly to keep her metabolism stoked and blood sugar levels steady. Here are some tips to tweak her daily menu.

EAT IN THE MORNING. Studies show that people who have breakfast are better able to lose weight and keep it off. "But one size doesn't always fit all," says Brooking. "Binges can be caused by so many things—stress, menstrual cycle, even genetics. If eating when she first wakes up causes Donna to overeat later, she can start her day with cappuccino, but then have a midmorning meal that combines a fiber and protein to help jump-start her metabolism and boost her energy."

CURB LIQUID CALORIES. Donna has 2 cups of cappuccino (each with 2 teaspoons of sugar) and 2 cups of tea (each with 2 teaspoons of honey). That's 150 calories in sweetener alone. Try smaller amounts, says Brooking, or a zero-calorie option, like Splenda, instead. She should also replace her wine or beer with flavored club soda or water a few nights a week.

KEEP SNACK PORTIONS IN CHECK. Nuts provide healthy fat, and prunes are packed with nutrients, but the combo is high in calories. "Donna's typical snack of seven walnuts and five prunes clocks in at 300 calories," says Blatner. She should pick one or the other and save her calories for real meals.

EXPAND MENU OPTIONS. "Different foods offer different nutritional profiles," says Brooking. "That's why variety is the central tenet of sound nutrition. Donna is in a rut. She eats the same thing day in and day out. But she can expand her choices and still create a healthy meal. Chicken, fish, and lean beef are all great protein foods."

The Sweet Tooth

"I lost 130 pounds but can't give up my chocolate."—Julia Griggs Havey, 47

If anyone knows the diet damage sugar can cause, it's Julia: She used to weigh 290, and chocolate and ice cream were mostly to blame. Then, 12 years ago, she shed

130 pounds by improving her diet and increasing her exercise. "I've written books about my weight loss and now coach others to live healthy," says Julia. "But in the past few years, I've put about 20 pounds back on, and I'm not happy about it." Julia still sticks to the habits that helped her lose: She drinks lots of water; gets her protein from chicken, fish, and egg whites; skips soda; watches her portions; and works out regularly.

"When I get busy, however, I have a tougher time eating healthy," she says. "I'll find myself giving in to my trigger foods more often. And if I'm not in bed by 11 p.m., I'm searching for a snack, which usually ends up being something sweet. My diet is always a work in progress, and right now, I know it needs a tweak."

EXPERT FIX: "Julia is savvy about weight loss," says Brooking. "She incorporates lots of steamed vegetables and fruit into her diet, which is great. But she does have a sweet tooth, and that's probably what's undoing her hard work." Some chocolate-covered almonds or a few handfuls of chocolate chips in the afternoon, cookies or sugary cereal after dinner—they all add up, says Blatner. To help curb her munchies, she should make sure each meal is well-balanced—3 ounces of protein, a cup or less of whole grains, and lots of vegetables. Here are some tips to get her back on track.

COOK IN BULK. "It's tough to find time to make meals every day, so when you do cook, prepare more than you need and freeze the extra portions," suggests Brooking. That way, even on the craziest days, you have a healthy home-cooked meal ready to reheat. And keep good-for-you snacks in the house, such as whole grain crackers or low-fat cheese wedges.

GET A LOWER-CALORIE CHOCOLATE FIX. Julia loves chocolate, but just five chocolate-covered almonds have 210 calories, and a giant soft-baked deli cookie could pack 400 to 500 calories. Try this instead, suggests Blatner: Drizzle fresh fruit with chocolate syrup (1 tablespoon is 54 calories), stir 1 tablespoon of chocolate chips (70 calories) into fat-free Greek-style yogurt, or sip diet hot chocolate (25 calories per packet).

HAVE PEPPERMINT AFTER DINNER. Because Julia is a classic night eater, she needs to find ways to tell her body the kitchen is closed, says Blatner. Chewing on peppermint-flavored gum and drinking peppermint tea are two great options: Researchers at Wheeling Jesuit University found that people who simply sniffed peppermint ate 23 percent fewer calories, on average, over a 5-day period.

YOU ASSUME CALORIES FROM HEALTHY, NATURAL FOODS ARE LOW

People consistently underestimate the calories in nutritious items such as yogurt, fish, and baked chicken, found researchers at Bowling Green State University who quizzed students on calorie counts.

"Just because a food is healthy doesn't mean you can eat big portions," says D. Milton Stokes, MPH, RD, owner of One Source Nutrition in Stamford, Connecticut. "A handful of nuts can be 200 calories or more. And if you add that without cutting back elsewhere, it could be the reason you're not losing weight."

Smarter move: Count all calories. Once you learn that ½ cup of cereal can have as much as 200 calories or that there are about 220 calories in that "single-serving" bottle of OJ, you'll be more prudent about how much you eat.

YOU EAT LIKE A BIRD FOR THE MONTH LEADING UP TO A BIG EVENT

Slashing significant calories might sound like the fast track to weight loss, but it's likely to backfire. In fact, nutrition experts recommend you don't dip below 1,200 to 1,500 calories a day.

"If you crash diet for more than 2 weeks or so, your metabolism will temporarily slow down," says Dr. Blackburn. "So the same exact dieting effort results in less and less weight loss."

SECRET TO EXTRA WEIGHT LOSS

Eat more fiber, say researchers at Brigham Young University. In a study of 252 women, those who ate 8 additional grams of total fiber for every 1,000 calories they consumed lost nearly 4½ pounds. Every gram decrease in total fiber intake resulted in an average weight gain of more than ½ pound.

To sneak in those extra grams of filling fiber daily, add a cup of raspberries to your yogurt or cereal, or toss ½ cup of lentils into your soup or salad.

BUFFET SECRETS OF THE NATURALLY SLIM

Serve-yourself smorgasbords, with their all-you-can-eat allure, are typically diet duds. But new research shows that there are fundamental differences between how overweight and healthy-weight people approach a spread. Their findings—based on behaviors at a Chinese food buffet—can help you stay on track when you're faced with the urge to graze.

LOOK BEFORE YOU EAT. 71 percent of normal-weight diners, versus 33 percent of obese people, browsed the food selections before serving themselves.

SIT IN A BOOTH. 38 percent of normal-weight diners sat in a booth instead of at a table (making it less convenient to get out), compared with 16 percent of obese diners.

PICK THE RIGHT CHAIR. 73 percent of normal-weight diners sat facing away from the buffet, versus 58 percent of obese people.

CHEW EACH BITE 15 TIMES. This was the average for normal-weight people. Obese diners chewed 12 times.

LEAVE LEFTOVERS ON YOUR PLATE. Normal-weight diners left just over a tenth of their food, while the obese eaters left about half that much.

The reason: Your body is conserving energy to keep you from losing weight too quickly. And that's not all. When you drastically cut calories, you lose muscle along with fat—especially if you haven't been exercising. Because muscle is your body's calorie-burning furnace, this can slow down your metabolism, even long after your crash diet is done.

Smarter move: Aim to shed about a pound a week. The slow, steady weight loss ensures you lose fat, not muscle.

"If you want to drop 10 pounds, get started 10 weeks before your goal, not 4," says Dr. Blackburn. "You'll have a better chance of actually taking off the weight permanently."

To drop a pound a week, shave 250 calories from your diet and burn an extra 250 calories through exercise each day. Visit www.prevention.com/myhealthtrackers to log your progress.

IS YOUR COOKBOOK MAKING YOU FAT?

Beware the creeping-calorie trend among time-tested recipes. When food scientists at Cornell University analyzed the 18 recipes that have appeared in every edition of *The Joy of Cooking*—the iconic cookbook that's been updated every 10 years since 1936—they found that the average calories per serving have increased nearly 63 percent. Even though the dishes—such as macaroni and cheese, chicken à la king, brownies, and apple pie—are essentially the same, richer ingredients and larger serving sizes have inflated calorie counts. To find healthy home-cooked meals that won't weigh you down, visit www.prevention.com/lowcal.

YOU SET SHORT-TERM WEIGHT-LOSS GOALS

The National Weight Control Registry (NWCR) estimates that only 20 percent of dieters successfully keep off lost weight for more than a year. That's because after we reach our goal, we let old eating habits creep back in. But people who win at weight loss consistently eat the same way even after they've slimmed down. In fact, the NWCR found that dieters who maintain their healthy eating habits every single day are 1½ times more likely to maintain their weight loss in the long run than those who relax their diets on the weekends.

Smarter move: Think of healthy eating as a work in progress, not as a "diet" with a beginning and an end. The key is making small changes you can maintain so they become long-term habits. Start by creating a list of problem areas in your diet, then tackle them one at a time. For example, if you snack on a heaping handful of Oreos every night before bed, set a goal of having two instead of six and cut back by one a day. Once you've made that a habit, pat yourself on the back and move on to your next goal.

YOUR SPLURGE FOODS ARE "LOW-FAT" AND "SUGAR-FREE"

Research suggests that when a food is described as a diet food, we're subconsciously primed to eat more—even if it's actually as caloric as regular food. When Cornell University researchers offered the same M&M's candies labeled either regular or low-fat to visitors at a university open house, visitors ate 28 percent more of the "low-fat" snacks. While less fat does not mean fewer calories, people make the assumption that it does, setting them up to overeat, say scientists.

Smarter move: First, check food labels. So-called diet foods frequently don't save you calories. Take low-fat chocolate chip cookies. Because they've been infused with extra carbs to add flavor, you save only 3 calories per cookie.

Once you have that reality check, follow the golden rule for any food: Keep close tabs on portions. Limit yourself to two small cookies, for example, or trade in a bowl of frozen yogurt for a kid's-size scoop. Measure out condiments such as low-fat sour cream or low-fat ranch dressing. And remember—if you prefer the flavor of full-fat foods, you'll still lose weight if you watch your portion sizes.

CHAPTER 8

New Food Flips for
WEIGHT LOSS

*Here's how to turn fat-promoting meals
into fat burners.*

Calorie-conscious eating doesn't mean boring eating. And it definitely doesn't mean forgoing foods you love. In fact, with our simple "food flips," everything you already eat can have a place in a healthy lifestyle.

So don't ditch your favorite fare, Instead, flip it! How does it work? Simply replace high-calorie and unhealthy ingredients with smarter items that taste just as delicious. Here's how to make over some popular dishes using a quick flip to these indulgent, down-home comfort foods. You'll be amazed how easy it is to lose weight without giving up taste or satisfaction—ever.

CAESAR SALAD

Flip out: Bottled Caesar dressing

Flip in: Simple homemade Caesar dressing

Calorie savings: 67

In a small bowl, whisk together $\frac{1}{4}$ cup pasteurized egg substitute; 1 clove garlic, minced; $1\frac{1}{2}$ teaspoons anchovy paste; $\frac{1}{2}$ teaspoon Dijon mustard; $\frac{1}{4}$ teaspoon Worcestershire sauce; and 2 tablespoons freshly squeezed lemon juice. Slowly add 2 tablespoons olive oil in a steady stream, whisking until combined. Stir in $\frac{1}{4}$ cup fresh Parmesan. Toss 8 cups coarsely torn romaine lettuce with dressing and $\frac{1}{2}$ cup croutons. Serves 4.

Caesar salad is famously fattening, and it's all the dressing's fault. Each 2-tablespoon portion of prepackaged Caesar dressing can contain 170 calories and 18 grams of fat. And who stops at only 2 tablespoons? Our quick-to-prepare homemade version slashes the amount of fat in half and does away with unnecessary ingredients such as high fructose corn syrup and sugar.

CANDIED SWEET POTATOES

Flip out: Brown sugar, marshmallows, butter

Flip in: Maple syrup, olive oil

Calorie savings: 93

Preheat the oven to 375°F. Wash and peel 4 medium sweet potatoes and cut into 1" pieces. Toss in a large bowl with 1 tablespoon olive oil, $\frac{1}{4}$ cup pure maple syrup, $\frac{1}{4}$ teaspoon salt, $\frac{1}{2}$ teaspoon cinnamon, a pinch of nutmeg, and $\frac{1}{4}$ cup chopped pecans. Place the mixture in a 13" x 9" baking dish and roast until fork-tender, about 40 minutes. Serves 4.

Traditional versions of this dish call for lots of brown sugar and a cup of marshmallows; no surprise it's called "candied." Plus, recipes are generally brimming with butter, which is laden with saturated fat. It's why a serving can pack in 430 calories. Our slimmed-down rendition is sweetened with just a touch of antioxidant-rich maple syrup and has the same nutty flavor but only 237 calories and 1 gram of saturated fat.

MACARONI AND CHEESE

Flip out: Powdered cheese, whole milk, butter

Flip in: Butternut squash, fat-free milk, reduced-fat Cheddar cheese

Calorie savings: 118

Prepare 8 ounces whole wheat rotini according to the package directions. In a medium saucepan, simmer $\frac{1}{2}$ cup fat-free milk with half of a 12-ounce package frozen butternut squash until combined. Remove from the heat and mix with 1 cup shredded reduced-fat Cheddar cheese, $\frac{1}{2}$ teaspoon salt, $\frac{1}{4}$ teaspoon dry mustard, and pepper to taste. Pour the drained pasta into an 8" x 8" baking dish, stir in the cheese mixture, and top with 1 tablespoon each Parmesan and bread crumbs. Bake at 375°F for 20 minutes. Serves 4.

Subbing in creamy butternut squash adds fiber and flavor, plus antioxidants that fight disease. Using fat-free milk and reduced-fat cheese, we lowered the calories per serving from 412 to 294, and unlike the boxed variety, our version has no artificial flavors. It also provides 45 percent of the daily recommendation for vision-protecting vitamin A.

PUMPKIN PIE

Flip out: Store-bought piecrust

Flip in: Quick graham cracker crust

Calorie savings: 175

Preheat the oven to 375°F and coat a 12-cup nonstick muffin pan with canola oil cooking spray. In a small bowl, combine 3 tablespoons wheat germ, 2 tablespoons ground flaxseed, and two $2\frac{1}{2}$" graham cracker squares, crushed. Add 1 heaping teaspoon of the mixture to each muffin cup. Whisk 2 large eggs and stir in one 15-ounce can plain pumpkin puree, one 12-ounce can fat-free evaporated milk, $\frac{2}{3}$ cup packed brown sugar, $1\frac{1}{2}$ teaspoons pumpkin pie spice, and 1 teaspoon vanilla extract. Pour evenly into cups. Bake for 30 to 35 minutes, or until sides are set and filling jiggles slightly. Mix $\frac{3}{4}$ cup nonfat Greek yogurt with $\frac{1}{4}$ cup pure maple syrup, then refrigerate. Let the pies rest 10 to 15 minutes before removing from the tins. Top each with a dollop of the maple-yogurt mixture. Serves 12.

Replacing the buttery crust with a thin layer of crushed graham crackers and nutty grains drops the calorie count from 316 to 141—without compromising flavor. Flaxseed adds heart- and brain-healthy omega-3s, while wheat germ boosts vitamin E, which helps control blood sugar. A piecrust that fights disease! What's not to love?

CREAMY TOMATO SOUP

Flip out: Heavy cream, regular chicken broth
Flip in: 2% milk, cannellini beans, low-sodium chicken broth
Calorie savings: 140

Combine two 14.5-ounce cans low-sodium chicken broth, one 28-ounce can crushed tomatoes, and several bay leaves in a medium saucepan over medium heat. In a small bowl, mash 1 cup rinsed and drained cannellini beans with the back of a spoon and set aside. When the soup bubbles, stir in 1 cup 2% milk and reduce the heat to low. Season to taste with a little salt and freshly ground black pepper and simmer for about 15 minutes, stirring occasionally. Remove and discard bay leaves and stir in the mashed beans. In small batches, puree the soup in a blender. Serves 4.

Traditional tomato soup gets its characteristic rich flavor and thick texture from heavy cream, which also boosts its calories. By using 2% milk instead of heavy cream, we nearly eliminated the soup's saturated fat content. The mashed beans do double duty: Their starches swell in the hot liquid, making the soup thick and hearty, and they boost the fiber. One serving supplies about one-quarter of your daily requirement. Switching from regular chicken broth to the reduced-fat, low-sodium type lowers sodium by 298 milligrams.

COSMOPOLITAN

Flip out: Store-bought Cosmopolitan mix
Flip in: Cranberry juice, fresh limes, agave nectar
Calorie savings: 91

Combine 1 ounce vodka with 1 teaspoon agave nectar, $\frac{1}{2}$ ounce fresh lime juice, and 1 ounce cranberry juice in a cocktail shaker. Add ice, shake, and garnish with a lime. Serves 1.

A drink made with sugary store-bought mix can contain 194 calories. Real fruit juice has no artificial colors and fewer calories, and it includes vitamins, antioxidants, and phytochemicals that boost health.

FROZEN MARGARITA

Flip out: Sugar-laden store-bought Margarita mix
Flip in: Zero-calorie mixers, fresh limes, agave nectar
Calorie savings: 160

Combine $\frac{1}{2}$ cup seltzer water with $\frac{1}{2}$ shot each tequila and triple sec, $\frac{1}{4}$ cup fresh lime juice, and 1 teaspoon agave nectar. Add ice, shake, and garnish with lime slices.

One frozen margarita made with store-bought mix can contain more than 300 calories. Swapping out the neon green concoction for fresh lime juice and agave nectar saves 160 calories.

ICE CREAM WITH STRAWBERRY TOPPING

Flip out: Hershey's strawberry syrup
Flip in: Strawberry compote
Calorie savings: 156

Warm 4 cups frozen strawberries with 2 tablespoons honey in a saucepan over medium heat until soft and tender. Let cool until the sauce thickens. Divide 2 cups vanilla ice cream into four bowls and top each with the strawberry compote. Serves 4.

Don't ditch ice cream entirely—just cut the portion down to $\frac{1}{2}$ cup from 1 cup, which slashes 137 calories. Replacing what's essentially strawberry-flavored high fructose corn syrup with a quick and easy compote supplies powerful disease-fighting antioxidants, 100 percent of your daily vitamin needs, and 4 grams of waist-friendly fiber.

FOODS NOT TO DITCH WHEN YOU DIET

You want to shed some pounds, and immediately your personal list of no-no's grows. No bread or potatoes—too many carbs. No chocolate—too fattening. Sound familiar?

Diets don't have to be so strict, says D. Milton Stokes, MPH, RD, owner of One Source Nutrition in Stamford, Connecticut. In fact, forbidding certain foods can backfire.

"Thanks to fad diets that aren't based in solid science, I often see clients avoiding foods that would help them control overeating or fight belly fat and ultimately lose weight," he says. "Worse still, having an off-limits list is like stuffing your cravings into a plastic bag. Eventually it's going to burst open, unleashing all your food urges at once, which leads to bingeing."

The real key to weight loss? "Mind your p's and q's—watch portions and choose quality, nutrient-rich foods," says Sari Greaves, RD, a national spokesperson for the American Dietetic Association. Here's how the top foods typically dismissed by dieters can help you happily slim down.

Bread

SLIM-DOWN EFFECT: Bread contains carbohydrates, which boost brain chemicals that curb overeating.

Bread is an excellent source of carbs, which your brain needs to produce serotonin, a neurotransmitter that promotes feelings of comfort and satisfaction, says Nina T. Frusztajer, MD, a Boston-based physician who specializes in nutrition and is coauthor of *The Serotonin Power Diet*.

"As your body digests carbohydrates, it releases insulin, which helps channel tryptophan, an amino acid, into the brain. Tryptophan then gets converted to serotonin," she explains.

When serotonin levels are optimal, you feel calm and happy and have fewer cravings; when they're low, you feel depressed and irritable, making you more likely to overeat. Breads containing whole grains are healthiest, and one serving equals one slice of bread, half an English muffin, or a small roll.

Pasta

SLIM-DOWN EFFECT: A high fluid content keeps you satisfied longer.

Cooked pasta and rice are about 70 percent water, and eating fluid-rich foods keeps you fuller longer, compared with dry foods, according to research from the British Nutrition Foundation. Like bread, the carbs in pasta boost serotonin to help curb overeating. The proper portion of pasta is ½ cup cooked, or about the size of an ice-cream scoop. Choose whole grain varieties for filling fiber, and add grilled chicken and lots of veggies to bulk up your dish even more.

Potatoes

SLIM-DOWN EFFECT: Forms resistant starch, a fiber that burns fat.

These veggies might be one of our most misunderstood foods. Fried or doused in sour cream, they're not going to help you lose weight. But when boiled or baked, a potato's starch absorbs water and swells. Once chilled, portions of the starch crystallize into a form that resists digestion—resistant starch. Unlike other types of fiber, resistant starch gets fermented in the large intestine, creating fatty acids that may block the body's ability to burn carbohydrates. In their place, you burn fat. A healthy potato serving is about the size of a fist.

Peanut Butter

SLIM-DOWN EFFECT: It's rich in healthy fats that help banish belly flab.

Studies show that diets high in monounsaturated fatty acids (abundant in peanut butter and nuts) prevent accumulation of fat around the midsection, boost calorie burn, and promote weight loss. In fact, women who eat one serving of nuts or peanut butter 2 or more times a week gain fewer pounds than women who rarely eat them, according to recent research from the Harvard School of Public Health.

One reason: A snack that includes peanut butter helps you stay full for up to 2½ hours, compared with 30 minutes for a carb-only snack such as a rice cake, finds research from Purdue University. (Carbohydrates satisfy a craving, while nuts keep you feeling full.) Peanut butter and nuts are high in calories, so stick with a 2-tablespoon portion, which is about the size of a golf ball.

(continued)

Cheese

SLIM-DOWN EFFECT: It's a great source of calcium, which burns calories.

At about 100 calories and 5 grams of fat per ounce, cheese usually tops the no-no list, but its calcium improves your ability to burn calories and fat, according to a recent research review. Not getting enough of this mineral might trigger the release of calcitriol, a hormone that causes the body to store fat.

Scientists at the University of Tennessee found that people on a reduced-calorie diet who included an extra 300 to 400 milligrams of calcium a day lost significantly more weight than those who ate the same number of calories but with less calcium. Scientists aren't exactly sure why, but eating calcium-rich foods is more effective than taking calcium supplements, and cheese has about 200 milligrams per ounce. Just stick to 2-ounce portions, and choose light varieties to get health benefits for half the calories.

Dark Chocolate

SLIM-DOWN EFFECT: It satisfies a common craving, preventing bingeing.

Up to 97 percent of women experience cravings, and chocolate is the most common and "intensely" craved food, according to a recent study. Having an occasional small serving of a favorite treat is better than depriving yourself, which may lead to a binge, says Greaves. In fact, people who tried not to think about chocolate ate two-thirds more of it than people who were told to talk about it freely, according to British research.

Dark varieties are more satisfying than milk chocolate, say scientists at the University of Copenhagen, but measure your portion and be mindful when you eat. Slowly savoring one or two squares of a high-quality dark chocolate bar will satisfy a craving more than wolfing down M&M's in front of the TV.

Fruit

SLIM-DOWN EFFECT: Fruit soothes a sweet tooth naturally for few calories.

Some dieters skip this low-calorie fare when they start watching the scale, thanks to once-popular diets that eliminated fruit in their most restrictive phases. But new research published in the journal *Obesity Reviews* looked at 16 different studies and found overwhelmingly that eating fruit is associated with weighing less.

In one study, women who added three small apples to their regular meals and snacks lost 2 pounds in 10 weeks without dieting. Although fruit does contain the natural sugar fructose, it doesn't raise blood sugar levels like table sugar does. Plus, it's high in water and filling fiber and low in calories. Aim to have three servings of fresh fruit daily, but skip the high-calorie juice. Great picks (with average calories per cup) include: fresh melon (50), grapes (60), berries (70), and citrus fruits (75).

CHAPTER 9

Stride Off Pounds
WITHOUT DIETING

Scientists discover the best way to walk off the weight.

Pop quiz: Two women go for a walk. One finishes quickly, the other takes her time. They each burn about 400 calories. So who sheds more belly fat? The obvious answer: It's a tie. But a surprising new study shows that the fast walker actually loses more. Researchers from the University of Virginia found that women who did three shorter, fast-paced walks a week (plus two longer, moderate-paced ones) lost 5 times more abdominal fat than those who simply strolled at a moderate speed 5 days a week, even though both groups burned exactly the same number of calories (400) per workout. The speedsters also dropped more than 2 inches from their waistlines, pared about 3 times more fat from their thighs, shed 4 times more total body fat, and lost almost 8 pounds over 16 weeks—all without dieting!

The improvements didn't stop there. The high-intensity exercisers lost about 3 times more visceral fat, which is the dangerous belly fat that wraps around organs such as the liver and kidneys and has been linked to diabetes, heart disease, and high blood pressure.

"Vigorous exercise raises levels of fat-burning hormones," says lead researcher Arthur Weltman, PhD, director of the exercise physiology laboratory at the university. It also increases afterburn (the number of calories your body uses postexercise as it recovers) by about 47 percent compared with lower-intensity workouts.

So how do you make all this science work for you? Start with our 8-week progressive walking plan, which includes both shorter, high-intensity workouts and longer, moderate-paced ones. Add in the Sculpting Moves to firm your ever-shrinking middle. In just 2 months, you could walk off one or two sizes—without dieting!

Then celebrate your success by walking a full or a half marathon. The 8-Week Plan will prime you for the challenge while flattening your belly, and our Walk-a-Marathon (or Half) Training will keep you on track to get in your best shape possible.

THE 8-WEEK PLAN

Workout at a Glance

Your goal: Walk 5 days a week, burning 400 calories each session, as they did in the study.

At least 3 days a week: Do a high-intensity Speed Walk.

At least 2 days a week: Do a lower-intensity Basic Walk.

Do the Sculpting Moves on any 3 nonconsecutive days of the week, working up to 2 sets by week 4.

Get started: To determine how long you need to walk to melt 400 calories, find your weight and walking speeds on the chart at right. The point at which they meet is your workout length. Note: The faster you walk or the heavier you are, the shorter your sessions will be, because you'll burn calories slightly faster.

WHAT HAPPY WALKERS DO

Brown Medical School scientists reviewed research on more than 2,300 exercisers. Here are their top stick-with-it strategies.

SPEED-DIAL SUPPORT. Motivating phone calls kept walkers accountable. Sign up for personalized workout reminders at extracon.com ($5 and up monthly after a free trial).

GET A DAILY DOSE. Don't let exercise be a 30-minutes-or-nothing endeavor. Even 10 minutes a day is enough to start a habit and get results.

SURF FOR ADVICE. Fitness-themed e-newsletters keep goals front and center, say researchers, while discussion forums give you 24–7 access to virtual workout buddies. Get both at www.prevention.com/walking.

WEIGHT	SPEED			
	3 MPH	**3.5 MPH**	**4 MPH**	**4.5 MPH**
140 lb	1 hr, 55 min	1 hr, 39 min	1 hr, 15 min	59 min
150	1 hr, 47 min	1 hr, 33 min	1 hr, 11 min	56 min
160	1 hr, 40 min	1 hr, 27 min	1 hr, 6 min	52 min
170	1 hr, 34 min	1 hr, 22 min	1 hr, 2 min	49 min
180	1 hr, 29 min	1 hr, 17 min	59 min	46 min
190	1 hr, 25 min	1 hr, 13 min	56 min	44 min
200	1 hr, 20 min	1 hr, 9 min	53 min	42 min
210	1 hr, 16 min	1 hr, 6 min	51 min	40 min
220	1 hr, 13 min	1 hr, 3 min	48 min	38 min

Tracey Staehle, a certified trainer in Simsbury, Connecticut, and creator of the *Walking Strong* DVD, designed the belly-sculpting workout. *Prevention* fitness director Michele Stanten created the marathon training plans.

To estimate your speed, time how quickly you can cover a mile* at both a Speed Walk pace (you can say a few words at a time but are mostly breathless) and a Basic Walk pace (you can talk but are slightly breathless). Based on your times, here's how fast you're walking:

20 minutes = 3 mph

17 minutes = 3.5 mph

15 minutes = 4 mph

13.5 minutes = 4.5 mph

Retest about every 2 weeks because you'll be able to walk faster as your fitness level improves.

* To calculate a mile, walk on a track (usually 4 laps) or treadmill; or use a pedometer (about 2,000 steps equals a mile), your car, or www.prevention.com/mywalkingmaps.

The Walks

SPEED WALK: 3 TIMES PER WEEK

For this routine, you want to push yourself. Try to go at a pace at which you are breathing heavily, but you can speak a couple of words at a time. (Back off if you can't.) Able to discuss dinner plans in detail? Go faster. Remember, everyone's idea of hard is different—for a beginner, 3 mph may be plenty, while someone who is very fit might need to push it to 4.5 mph or more to get results.

To help you get up to speed, take short breaks by slowing to a moderate pace. As you progress, do this recovery less frequently until you're able to keep up the pace for the full hour or more.

Take a 1-minute break (that is, a moderate pace):

Week 1: Every 5 minutes

Week 2: Every 10 minutes

Week 3: Every 15 minutes

Week 4: After 20 minutes; repeat if needed

Week 5: After 30 minutes; repeat if needed

Week 6: After 40 minutes; repeat if needed

Week 7: After 50 minutes

Week 8: Walk for 60 minutes (or the duration of the workout) at a high intensity, without taking a break.

BASIC WALK: 2 TIMES PER WEEK

Walk at a moderate (somewhat challenging) pace. You could easily discuss the latest episode of your favorite show, but need to pause between phrases to catch your breath. Because you'll be going slower, you'll have to walk a little longer than you do in the Speed Workout in order to burn 400 calories. (See the speed chart on page 85 to determine how long you need.) Can't spare that much time all at once? You can divide your workouts into smaller chunks, such as three 20- to 30-minute sessions, and still get the same results, says Dr. Weltman.

For all walks, go at an easy pace for 3 to 5 minutes to warm up and cool down.

THE SCULPTING MOVES: 3 TIMES PER WEEK

WALKING A MARATHON (OR HALF) TAUGHT ME . . .

NOT TO SHY AWAY FROM A CHALLENGE. "The training has given me more self-discipline and convinced me that other things in life probably aren't as bad as they first seem, either. It also reminded me that I actually like being outside; how good it feels to breathe deep, relaxed breaths; and that sweating is quite nice when accompanied by a feeling of accomplishment."

—Lisa Hollingsworth, 40, Washington, DC

WALKERS ARE ATHLETES, TOO! "Sometimes I felt silly mentioning what I was working toward, especially around 'real' athletes, because I was only doing half of the marathon and only walking it. But when I crossed the finish line and received my medal and blanket just like the runners, I knew I deserved to be there, too. Next year, I plan to walk the half again—only faster!"

—Anne Reilly, 46, Lancaster, Pennsylvania

DOING SOMETHING FOR MYSELF IS GOOD FOR MY FAMILY! "The guilt I felt over not spending all my time with my family was completely unfounded. My 5-year-old son, Jacob, told his class that I was in a race and was going to win a gold medal. When I showed him my medal, he held it as if it were the most precious thing in the world and said, 'I love you, Mom. You're my hero.'"

—Rebecca Renicker, 33, Dover, Ohio

I WANT TO BE FIT, NOT SKINNY. "I am in the best shape of my life, even though I am still overweight. I've lost 48 pounds so far, I've increased my endurance, and I look more toned than ever before."

—Pamela McNab, 45, Fredericksburg, Virginia

YOU'RE NEVER TOO OLD. "Walking marathons keeps my fitness program fresh. Turns out I can do a lot more than I thought I could. I did my first marathon at age 73 and completed my third last November on my 75th birthday, each with one of my three children."

—Sara Burneson, 75, Westlake, Ohio

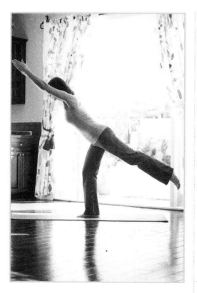

< BALANCE EXTENSION

FIRMS DEEP AND FRONT ABS

Stand tall, pull abs in, and raise left knee toward chest, grasping shin with hands. Release and swing leg behind you, toes pointed, as upper body tilts forward, arms extended. Keep abs tight and supporting knee slightly bent. Your arms, torso, and leg should be aligned. Hold for 1 count; bring knee to chest again and repeat. Do 6 to 8 reps, then switch legs.

MAKE IT EASIER: Tap toes to floor behind you instead of lifting leg.

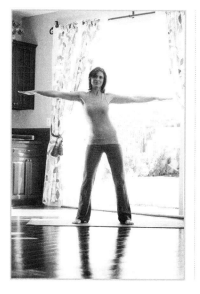

< SIDE-TO-SIDE REACH

FIRMS DEEP AND FRONT ABS

Stand with arms extended at shoulder height, palms down. Keeping hips still, lift rib cage and slide it side to side (that's 1 rep), as if your body were in a tug-of-war. Do 16 reps.

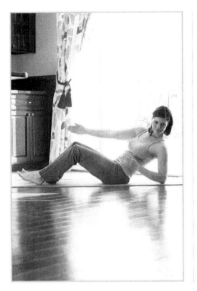

⊙ ELBOW TAP BACK

FIRMS DEEP, FRONT, AND SIDE ABS

Sit with knees bent, heels on floor, arms extended, and torso at about a 45-degree angle to floor. Keeping abs tight, rotate torso to left as you pull left arm back, tapping elbow to floor. Return to center. Do 8 to 10 reps; repeat to right side.

MAKE IT EASIER: Don't lean back as far; rotate torso without tapping elbow to floor.

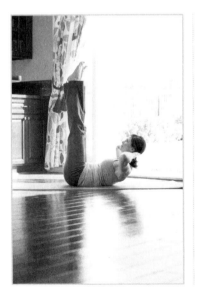

⊙ NARROW/WIDE CRUNCH

FIRMS FRONT ABS

Lie faceup, legs extended above hips, hands behind head. Lift head, neck, and shoulders toward knees. As you lower, open legs into a wide V. Repeat, bringing legs together as you lift. Do 10 to 12 reps.

MAKE IT EASIER: Don't crunch up as high or lower legs as wide.

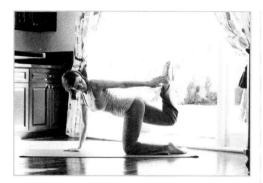

◉ POINTER REACH

FIRMS DEEP, FRONT, AND SIDE ABS; LOWER BACK; HAMSTRINGS

Begin on all fours, knees under hips and palms under shoulders. Extend left arm forward at shoulder height while lifting right leg behind you, abs tight. Reach left arm behind you and bend right leg to touch sole of foot. Do 10 to 12 reps; switch sides.

MAKE IT EASIER: Lower back leg to floor and just reach arm behind you without touching foot.

YES, YOU CAN WALK A MARATHON

Thousands of readers, most of them beginners, already have done it—and many keep coming back for more! Some have even completed over a dozen events since joining Team Prevention in 2005, which participants say leaves them with boundless confidence; a stronger, fitter body; and newfound friendships. So join the fun!

Team Prevention will be with you every step of the way, from picking the right training sneakers to receiving your medal at the finish line. Let us help you turn walking into a life- and body-changing experience. To register, learn more, or just get tips to train for an event of your choice, go to www. prevention. com/team. Here are some benefits of joining.

- Follow a walking calendar that offers daily tips.
- Map your routes and calculate your calorie burn.
- Chat with other readers-in-training.
- Ask our walking coach all your burning questions.
- Get expert advice from top docs, dietitians, and trainers.
- Meet our mentors, who will keep you motivated.

YOU CAN DO IT! HERE'S HOW

The following training schedules are perfect for experienced walkers—anyone, for example, who has just completed the 8-Week Plan or has been exercising regularly for 6 weeks or more and can walk for at least 60 minutes at a time. If you're just getting started, find expanded training plans for your level at www.prevention.com/team.

Half Marathon Training

WEEK	SUNDAY	MONDAY	TUESDAY	WEDNESDAY	THURSDAY	FRIDAY	SATURDAY
1	M: 60 min	Xtrain	I: 45 min	Rest	M: 60 min	Xtrain	E: 6 miles (about 1.5–2 hr)
2	R: 30 min	Xtrain	I: 45 min	Rest	M: 60 min	Xtrain	E: 7 miles (about 1.75–2.5 hr)
3	R: 30 min	Xtrain	I: 45 min	Rest	M: 60 min	Xtrain	E: 8 miles (about 2–2.75 hr)
4	R: 30 min	Xtrain	I: 45 min	Rest	M: 60 min	Xtrain	E: 9 miles (about 2.25–3.25 hr)
5	R: 30 min	Xtrain	I: 45 min	Rest	M: 60 min	Xtrain	E: 10 miles (about 2.5–3.5 hr)
6	R: 30 min	Xtrain	I: 30 min	Rest	M: 45 min	Xtrain	E: 5 miles (about 1.25–1.75 hr)
7	R: 30 min	M: 30 min	R: 30 min	Rest	M: 30 min	Rest	R: 20 min You're ready to race!

Your Key

Moderate Walk (M): Maintain a brisk pace, as if you need to get to an appointment.

Cross-Train (Xtrain): To prevent burnout and injury, do an activity that's different from walking, such as strength training, yoga, Pilates, swimming, or cycling. Keep the intensity moderate, and aim for about 20 to 30 minutes.

Intensity Walk (I): Shoot for a vigorous pace the entire time, or alternate short bursts of speed (30 to 60 seconds) with equal intervals of brisk walking (see Moderate Walk). As you become more fit, increase the length of the speed

Full Marathon Training

WEEK	SUNDAY	MONDAY	TUESDAY	WEDNESDAY	THURSDAY	FRIDAY	SATURDAY
1	M: 60 min	Xtrain	I: 45 min	Rest	M: 60 min	Xtrain	E: 6 miles (about 1.5–2 hr)
2	R: 30 min	Xtrain	I: 45 min	Rest	M: 60 min	Xtrain	E: 8 miles (about 2–2.75 hr)
3	R: 30 min	Xtrain	I: 45 min	Rest	M: 60 min	Xtrain	E: 10 miles (about 2.5–3.5 hr)
4	R: 30 min	Xtrain	I: 45 min	Rest	M: 60 min	Xtrain	E: 12 miles (about 3–4.25 hr)
5	R: 30 min	Xtrain	I: 60 min	Rest	M: 75 min	Xtrain	E: 7 miles (about 1.75–2.5 hr)
6	R: 30 min	Xtrain	I: 60 min	Rest	M: 75 min	Xtrain	E: 14 miles (about 3.5–4.75 hr)
7	R: 30 min	Xtrain	I: 60 min	Rest	M: 90 min	Xtrain	E: 16 miles (about 4–5.5 hr)
8	R: 30 min	Xtrain	I: 60 min	Rest	M: 90 min	Xtrain	E: 18 miles (about 4.5–6 hr)
9	R: 30 min	Xtrain	I: 60 min	Rest	M: 75 min	Xtrain	E: 20 miles (about 5–7 hr)
10	R: 30 min	Xtrain	I: 60 min	Rest	M: 60 min	Xtrain	E: 10 miles (about 2.5–3.5 hr)
11	R: 30 min	Xtrain	I: 45 min	Rest	M: 45 min	Xtrain	E: 5 miles (about 1.25–1.75 hr)
12	R: 30 min	M: 30 min	R: 30 min	Rest	M: 30 min	Rest	R: 20 min You're ready to race!

bouts until you can maintain the faster pace for the duration of the workout. This type of training will increase your speed.

Endurance Walk (E): Go at a slightly slower pace than a Moderate Walk but faster than a Recovery Walk. Distance, not speed, is the key here.

Recovery Walk (R): To loosen up from the previous day's long workout or rest up before the big event, stroll at an easy pace.

CHAPTER 10

The New-Science, NEW-YOU WORKOUT

Shrink a size in 14 days! Your super shape-up starts now!

This revolutionary, science-backed workout is reader tested and can help you shed up to 12 pounds and 22 inches in just 2 weeks. Intrigued by research spotlighting eccentric training as one of the most effective ways to get firm, we asked fitness expert Chris Freytag to create a superfast shape-up program using this unique technique. When we put a group of readers on the plan, the results were eye-popping: Testers lost an average of 6 pounds and 10 inches in 14 days, with the most successful volunteers losing up to 12 pounds and more than 22 inches all over.

The secret is in the program's slow-motion strength routine. Instead of lifting and lowering for 2 counts each, you'll double the lengthening "eccentric" phase of an exercise (for example, straightening your arm during a biceps curl) to 4 counts.

"Each muscle fiber works harder so you get firmer faster," explains Freytag.

An East Carolina University study found that women who did eccentric training increased their strength nearly twice as much as those who lifted weights at a normal pace after just 1 week. You'll also build more muscle and rev up your metabolism to burn fat faster.

Get started today with our exclusive jump-start plan that will help you shed pounds, shrink inches, and feel confident in just 14 days! It's been adapted from *2-Week Total Body Turnaround* by Chris Freytag with Alyssa Shaffer and the editors of *Prevention* (Rodale, 2009).

WORKOUT AT A GLANCE

The Strength Plan

What you'll need: 2 sets of dumbbells (2 to 5 and 8 to 10 pounds); a chair.

Week 1: Do the routine 6 days a week, alternating between Workout A (for your chest, back, and abs) and Workout B (for your arms, legs, and butt).

Week 2: Follow the same schedule, but challenge yourself by trying the "make it harder" options.

OUR EXPERT

American Council on Exercise board member Chris Freytag is the author of *2-Week Total Body Turnaround*, creator of its companion DVDs, and model for the workouts here, which she designed.

The Cardio Plan

Weeks 1 and 2: Walk for 30 minutes 6 days a week, alternating between the Speed Ladder interval routine and Power Walk workout on page 103.

To rev up results: Follow a healthy diet of about 1,600 calories a day.

Your 2-Week Turnaround

Day 1	Strength Plan A; Speed Ladder
Day 2	Strength Plan B; Power Walk
Day 3	Strength Plan A; Speed Ladder
Day 4	Strength Plan B; Power Walk
Day 5	Strength Plan A; Speed Ladder
Day 6	Strength Plan B; Power Walk
Day 7	Active rest (no formal workout, but keep moving throughout the day)
Day 8	Strength Plan A with Make It Harder options; Speed Ladder
Day 9	Strength Plan B with Make It Harder options; Power Walk
Day 10	Strength Plan A with Make It Harder options; Speed Ladder
Day 11	Active rest
Day 12	Strength Plan B with Make It Harder options; Power Walk
Day 13	Strength Plan A with Make It Harder options; Speed Ladder
Day 14	Strength Plan B with Make It Harder options; Power Walk

For continued success, repeat or modify to alternate cardio and strength workouts.

THE STRENGTH PLAN: WORKOUT A

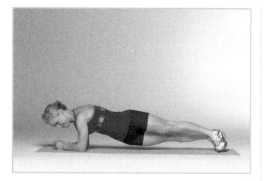

⊗ HIP DROP

FIRMS FRONT AND SIDE ABS

Lie facedown, balancing on elbows, forearms, and toes; abs tight. Slow it down: Twist to right and lower right hip to floor in 4 counts. (Keep back straight.) Raise to start position in 2 counts. Repeat to left. Do 8 to 10 times each side.

MAKE IT HARDER (WEEK 2): Do 12 to 15 times each side.

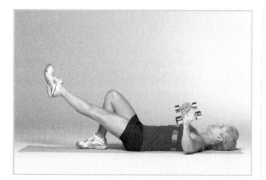

⊗ BEACH BALL HUG

FIRMS CHEST, ABS, HIPS

Lie faceup, dumbbells above chest, elbows slightly bent, palms in. Raise left leg so shin is parallel to floor. Slow it down: Lower arms out to sides in 4 counts as you straighten left leg, keeping foot off the floor. In 2 counts, pull knee back in and raise arms, squeezing chest muscles as if you're hugging a beach ball. Do 6 times; repeat with right leg.

MAKE IT HARDER (WEEK 2): Raise both feet off the floor.

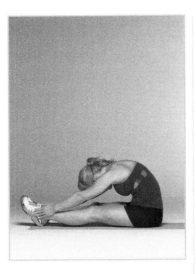

< FULL-BODY ROLL-UP

FIRMS ABS

Lie faceup, legs extended, arms overhead, palms facing each other. Raise arms toward feet; pull abs in; roll head, shoulders, and back off the floor; and reach toward toes in 4 counts.

SLOW IT DOWN: Roll back down to floor one vertebrae at a time, taking about 6 to 8 counts to lower.

MAKE IT HARDER (WEEK 2): Hold a light weight (2 to 3 pounds) in both hands.

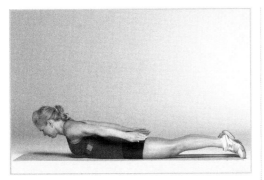

< BREAST STROKE

FIRMS UPPER AND MIDDLE BACK

Lie facedown, arms extended overhead, palms facing in. Lift head and arms off the floor and hold for 2 counts. Lift chest a few inches off the floor and swim arms out to sides and down toward legs (thumbs toward floor) in 2 counts. (Keep abs tight, toes on floor.)

SLOW IT DOWN: Lower chest and bend arms, bringing them along body back to start position in 4 counts. Do 8 to 10 times.

MAKE IT HARDER (WEEK 2): As you lift chest and swim arms, raise both feet off the floor, then lower.

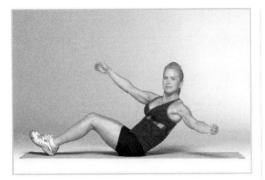

⊘ READ THE PAPER

FIRMS FRONT AND SIDE ABS

Sit with knees bent, heels on the floor, arms in front of body, as if holding a closed newspaper. **SLOW IT DOWN:** Roll back halfway down to the floor and twist to left in 4 counts, as if opening the paper on left side. Pull yourself up to start position in 2 counts. Repeat on right side. Do 8–12 times per side.

MAKE IT HARDER (WEEK 2): Hold a light weight (2 to 3 pounds) in each hand.

THE STRENGTH PLAN: WORKOUT B

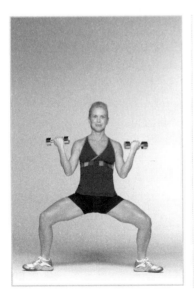

⊘ PLIÉ WITH BICEPS CURL

FIRMS BICEPS, GLUTES, QUADS, INNER THIGHS

Stand with feet wide, toes out, dumbbells by thighs, palms forward. Bend knees and lower for 2 counts, as you curl weights toward shoulders. **SLOW IT DOWN:** Squeeze glutes and inner thighs as you stand up and straighten arms in 4 counts. Do 8 to 12 times.

MAKE IT HARDER (WEEK 2): Use heavier weights.

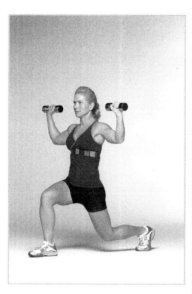

< FORWARD LUNGE AND RAISE THE ROOF

FIRMS SHOULDERS, CORE, BUTT, QUADS

Stand with feet together, dumbbells overhead, palms forward.

SLOW IT DOWN: Step right foot forward and bend both knees as you lower weights toward shoulders in 4 counts. (Keep right knee over ankle.) Stand up to start position, pressing weights overhead in 2 counts. Do 8 to 12 times; switch legs.

MAKE IT HARDER (WEEK 2): Swing left knee forward to hip height as you stand up.

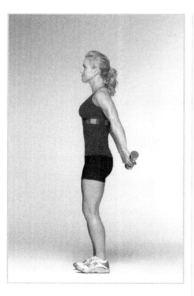

< SQUAT WITH STRAIGHT-ARM PRESSBACK

FIRMS SHOULDERS, ARMS, GLUTES, QUADS

Stand with feet about 4 inches apart, dumbbells at sides, palms facing behind you.

SLOW IT DOWN: Sit back, keeping weight over heels, as arms swing forward toward knees for 4 counts. Stand up in 2 counts while pressing weights behind you. Do 8 to 12 times.

MAKE IT HARDER (WEEK 2): Lift left leg back and squeeze glutes as you stand; switch legs halfway through set.

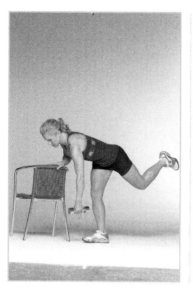

⊙ TIP IT OVER

FIRMS ARMS, BUTT, HAMSTRINGS

Stand with dumbbell in left hand at side, right hand on chair for balance.

SLOW IT DOWN: Keeping spine straight and abs tight, lean forward in 4 counts, and lower left arm while lifting left leg. Stand up in 2 counts, while doing a biceps curl and raising left knee in front. Do 8 times; switch sides.

MAKE IT HARDER (WEEK 2): Use a heavier weight and skip the chair.

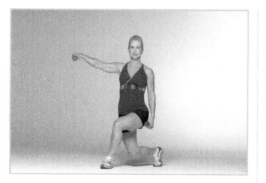

⊙ CURTSY LAT RAISE

FIRMS SHOULDERS, BUTT, OUTER THIGHS, QUADS

Stand with feet together, dumbbells at sides, palms in.

SLOW IT DOWN: Cross right leg behind left, bend knees, and lower as you raise right arm out to side in 4 counts. (Keep left knee over ankle and facing forward.) Stand up to start position and lower arm in 2 counts. Do 8 to 12 times; switch sides.

MAKE IT HARDER (WEEK 2): As you stand up, lift right leg out to side.

THE CARDIO PLANS

Speed Ladder

This challenging workout features intervals that get increasingly hard but shorter, followed by brief recovery periods.

TIME	ACTIVITY (SPEED*)	INTENSITY**	HOW IT FEELS
0:00	Warmup (3.0 mph)	4	Breathing harder; can speak in full sentences
4:00	Moderate walk (3.5 mph)	5	Slightly breathless; can still speak in full sentences
9:00	Brisk walk (3.75 mph)	6	Somewhat breathless; can speak in short sentences only
13:00	Moderate walk (3.5 mph)	5	
15:00	Power walk (4.0 mph)	7	Mostly breathless; can speak in phrases only
18:00	Moderate walk (3.5 mph)	5	
20:00	Fast walk (4.5 mph)	8	Breathless; can speak just a few words at a time
22:00	Moderate walk (3.5 mph)	5	
24:00	Speed walk or jog (5.0 mph)	9	Very breathless; can't speak
25:00	Cooldown (3.0 mph)	4	Breathing slows
30:00	Finished		

*These are suggested speeds only and may not be appropriate for everyone. The right speed for you should be based on intensity recommendations and how you feel.

**Based on a 1-to-10 scale, with 1 being extremely easy and 10 so hard that you can't sustain the pace for more than a few seconds.

Power Walk

This cardio routine is a great way to build endurance while burning calories.

TIME	ACTIVITY (SPEED*)	INTENSITY**	HOW IT FEELS
0:00	Warmup (3.0 mph)	4	Breathing harder; can speak in full sentences
5:00	Power walk (3.5–4.0 mph)	5–7	Somewhat breathless; can speak in short sentences only
25:00	Cooldown (3.0 mph)	4	Breathing slows
30:00	Finished		

SUCCESS STORIES

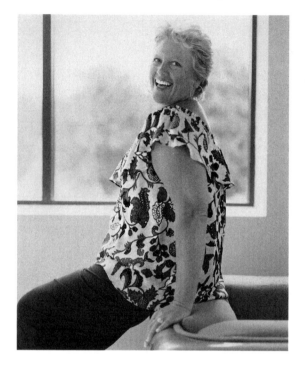

"I've lost 55 pounds in 7 months!"

—Teresa McDonald, 48

2-WEEK RESULTS: Lost 11 pounds, 10¾ inches (2 off waist)

A serious car accident left McDonald with back problems, and raising two daughters gave her little time for exercise. As a result, her weight crept up to almost 250 pounds. "My father died of a heart attack. I want to be sure I'm around for my kids."

BIGGEST SURPRISE: "I used to truly hate exercise; now I crave it. If I go a day without doing something, I feel sluggish and tired. On days when I'm not motivated, I think of the results I've had, and it gets me going."

BIGGEST SUCCESS: "I went from a size 24 to a size 14 in 6 months, and I'm still losing! Plus, my back pain is gone."

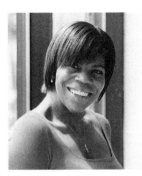

"I flattened my belly and got energized!"
—Linda Agnes, 41

2-WEEK RESULTS: Lost 12 pounds, 16 inches (4½ off waist)

Agnes used to run or lift weights 6 days a week. But after a hysterectomy 3 years ago, followed by hip surgery a year later, her activity level plummeted and she gained more than 40 pounds. "I was exhausted. Every night, I'd come home from work and just sack out on the couch. I couldn't move."

BIGGEST SURPRISE: "My joints used to hurt all the time. Now it feels really good to move, and I won't need to have another hip operation!"

BIGGEST SUCCESS: "I dropped more than 8 pounds in 7 days. After 2 weeks, my stomach looked significantly flatter. Six months later, I'm down about 20 pounds."

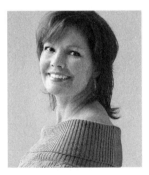

"I dropped nearly a dozen inches."
—Michele Knapek, 47

2-WEEK RESULTS: Lost 6 pounds, 11¾ inches (3 off waist)

Since hitting perimenopause, Knapek noticed that losing weight was getting increasingly difficult, despite biking and walking regularly. "My daughter's wedding was coming up in a few months. I really wanted to lose a few pounds, but the scale was stuck."

BIGGEST SURPRISE: "All of those miserable perimenopausal symptoms—sleepless nights, headaches, bloating—went away almost completely!"

BIGGEST SUCCESS: "My arms were more defined, and my belly looked flatter. I reshaped my body, and I didn't even have to put on Spanx for the wedding!"

CHAPTER 11

The Plateau
BUSTER

Our experts helped three women get the scale moving and drop their most stubborn fat.

You ate better, exercised more, and watched with joy as your efforts were reflected in the descending numbers on the scale—until, that is, the scale just stopped. A weight loss plateau is undeniably frustrating, but it's also normal.

In an analysis of 80 studies on dieters, researchers found that weight loss typically halts after 6 months, according to a report in the *Journal of the American Dietetic Association*. And that stall can last weeks, months, or even longer.

The solution: We asked a team of experts—a nutritionist, a certified personal trainer, and a psychologist—to work with three women for 8 weeks to get the scale moving again fast. The experts pored over the women's diets, exercise regimens, everyday habits, and attitudes, then offered adjustments to their routines and new strategies to help them restart their fat-burning engines. Their advice can help you reach your weight loss goals, too.

The following experts coached the women through their lifestyle makeovers.

DIET: Lisa R. Young, PhD, RD, adjunct professor of nutrition at New York University and author of *The Portion Teller Plan: The No-Diet Reality Guide to Eating, Cheating, and Losing Weight Permanently*

EXERCISE: Chris Freytag, personal trainer, creator of more than a dozen fitness DVDs, and author of four books, including *2-Week Total Body Turnaround*

ATTITUDE: Ann Kearney-Cooke, PhD, psychologist specializing in body image, emotional eating, and weight and author of *Change Your Mind, Change Your Body*

. . . .

CHRISSY BRENNAN, 44

"I BROKE A 4-YEAR WEIGHT LOSS STALL!"

A three-time New York City marathoner, Chrissy Brennan now finds it hard to remember the accomplished runner she once was. Her recent attempts at exercise and eating right are erratic, frequently falling victim to the long days at her high-stress marketing job. Having worked at health and fitness magazines for nearly a decade prior, Chrissy is well-versed in weight loss: She's read the science on exercise and knows how to incorporate healthy foods—yet she's often overcome by cravings, especially at night. The result: a creeping gain of about 20 pounds and a years-long plateau.

Expert Strategies

DIET

"Chrissy eats pretty well during the day, but after work her diet falls apart," says Lisa R. Young, PhD, RD. "She gets home late and grabs whatever is in arm's reach." To help break that pattern, follow these guidelines.

Eat real meals. Like many dieters, Chrissy tries to save calories by having a handful of crackers and cheese for lunch.

"But a big salad with 3 ounces of chicken and a small whole wheat roll is more filling and more nutritious and has about as many calories," says

Dr. Young. Also, having a more satisfying breakfast and lunch will help prevent overeating at night.

Prepare reheatable foods. It's tough to cook when it's late, so Chrissy should make a batch of grilled chicken on the weekend so she has lean protein ready to go. Other simple staples: frozen vegetables, instant brown rice, and figure-friendly frozen fruit or fudge pops to satisfy a sweets craving.

EXERCISE

Chrissy has time to work out only in the mornings and sometimes can't get herself going. But to jump-start weight loss, she needs 4 or 5 days of cardio sessions and two or three strength-training workouts every week. Here's how she should stay motivated.

Vary each workout. She can go running one day, walking or biking the next; when she doesn't feel like heading out, she can pop in a workout DVD.

Keep track. She should write down how many minutes, miles, and sets. A journal will keep her more accountable and therefore more likely to follow through, says personal trainer Chris Freytag.

ATTITUDE

A cookie might make a stressful day feel brighter, but before giving in, Chrissy should practice being mindful of her decisions so she avoids making bad ones, says Ann Kearney-Cooke, PhD. Here's how.

Ride out a craving. Hold off a little before indulging. If she still wants the cookie after 15 minutes, she should have it. But waiting helps develop the capacity to delay gratification, and that's key to success.

Her Results

Lost 11 pounds and ½ inch off waist

"Stocking up on easy-prep meals made a difference in my diet. Lentil soup and veggie burgers are my go-to dinners, and while I admit I wasn't excited about frozen fruit pops for dessert, they do satisfy my cravings well enough. What I did love right away was working out with DVDs. Doing so helped get me back in the habit of regular exercise. I feel more balanced now, and I'm thrilled with the results."

DONNA COULSON, 61

"I SHED 2½ INCHES FROM MY MIDDLE!"

After hovering at around 145 pounds for the better part of a decade, Donna Coulson upped her exercise, trimmed her portions, and dropped 10 pounds of the 15 that is her goal—and then the scale got stuck. Part of the reason, she believes, is her jam-packed schedule.

As a self-employed career coach and professional speaker, Donna travels often and works long hours, which takes a toll on her energy levels and eating habits. Though she tried subbing more salads and soups into her diet and squeezing in workouts as best she could, her weight hadn't budged for 3 months.

Expert Strategies

DIET

Donna tends to skip lunch, then overeat at her frequent client dinners. Nibbling a few ounces of cheese beforehand can help control her hunger, says Dr. Young. Metabolism also slows as we age; to keep hers revved, Donna should stick to a three-meal, two-snack day and try these tips to keep calories in check.

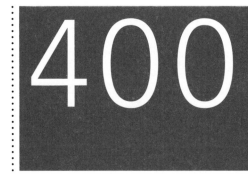

400
CALORIES BURNED IN 2 HOURS OF BOWLING, COMPARED WITH 68 BURNED WATCHING A MOVIE, ACCORDING TO THE SCHOOL OF PUBLIC HEALTH OF THE UNIVERSITY OF SOUTH CAROLINA

Work fiber and protein into every meal. Both help regulate blood sugar and keep you feeling fuller longer. Donna can add a few nuts to her cereal, opt for fiber-rich bean soup, and toss tuna in her salad.

Swap in low-calorie sweets. Donna loves Mallomars, but one serving has 120 calories. Young suggests Donna try meringue-type cookies, which have the same light texture but fewer calories, or have one or two Hershey's Kisses (about 20 calories each).

EXERCISE

Every weekend, Donna logs 6 miles with her walking club, and she tries to hit the weight machines a few days a week. Her consistency is good, says Freytag, but to see more results, she needs to try these tips.

Pick up the pace. Donna strolls when she walks, which is great for socializing but not for fat burning, says Freytag. Adding intervals can burn more calories, and studies show it also helps shrink more belly fat.

Do Pilates once a week. "The risk of injury from a fall increases as we get older," explains Freytag. It's important that Donna add core-building and flexibility workouts to her regimen to improve her balance.

ATTITUDE

Donna gives tirelessly to everyone in her life, but to sustain weight loss, you have to make yourself a priority. Here's how to stay focused.

Set aside 75 minutes a day for health. That's about how much time most people need to follow a weight-loss plan, says Dr. Kearney-Cooke. "Make a pie chart of how you spend your time now. Then make another chart that allots 45 minutes for exercise, 15 minutes for relaxation, and 15 more for food prep."

Her Results

Lost 4 pounds and 2½ inches off waist

"I learned that if you do what you've always done, you'll get what you've always gotten. Now I walk faster, lift more weight, and do Pilates. I miss my Mallomars, but when I crave chocolate, I'll have an apple, then a Hershey's Kiss, and

THE STUCK-SCALE SOLUTION

Keeping off pounds during the winter might be as easy as avoiding the couch on the weekends, say Vanderbilt University Medical Center researchers. Their new study found that women moved the least in December, January, and February, translating to a 10 percent drop in calorie burn compared with the summer months. The biggest culprit: lounging around on the weekends, which resulted in a 100-calorie surplus. Here are 10 fun cold-weather ways to torch those 100 calories fast.

1. Snowshoe for 11 minutes.
2. Ice-skate for 13 minutes.
3. Go sledding for 13 minutes (walk up the hill).
4. Shovel snow from your driveway for 15 minutes.
5. Splash around an indoor pool for 15 minutes.
6. Walk laps around the mall for 18 minutes.
7. Have a snowball fight for 19 minutes.
8. Dance for 20 minutes.
9. Build a snowman for 22 minutes.
10. Go bowling for 30 minutes.

that does the trick. Though I'm still pretty busy, I am more committed to me: I exercise before work and pack a snack before every late-night event. I have more energy, I dropped two sizes, and I'm still losing weight!"

LISA SPODAK, 39
"I LOST 60 POUNDS, THEN LOST 10 MORE!"

Last year, Lisa Spodak shed 60 pounds with exercise and Weight Watchers—but then losing got harder. For months, she dropped and regained the same few pounds, with much frustration. Lisa has struggled with her size for more than 25 years, since she was in her early teens. She's lost similar amounts of weight in the past, but when she hit a plateau, she gave up and put it all back on. This time, she's hoping to break the pattern and keep the scale moving.

Expert Strategies

DIET

Lisa steams veggies, grills chicken, and skips alcohol, which are all good, healthy habits. But her seemingly inconsequential choices might be stalling her success, says Dr. Young. The following diet tweaks will help.

Limit starch to one meal and snack per day. Lisa might have cereal for breakfast, a sandwich for lunch, crackers as a snack, and pasta at night. That's 5 servings of starch.

"Consider your daily menu," says Dr. Young. "If pasta is for dinner, have salad for lunch."

Visualize proper portions. Lisa puts cheese on sandwiches and enjoys macaroni or meat for dinner, which are all fine choices, in the right amounts: A serving of cheese looks like three dominoes; ½ cup of pasta, half a baseball; and 3 ounces of meat, a deck of cards.

EXERCISE

She walks 3 days a week, strength-trains twice, and on Saturdays takes classes at the gym. That helped her lose the first 60 pounds; but to rev her fat-burn, she has to up the intensity. Here's how.

Use a heart rate monitor for cardio. It tells you if you're burning maximum calories. (To determine your target, go to www.prevention.com/heartrate.) Lisa can also tell she's working out hard enough if she's breathing through her mouth and sweating lightly.

Strength-train for 1 hour a week. That can be divided into three 20-minute sessions, with moves that target the arms, back, and legs in each. Lisa should aim for 3 sets of 15 reps; if her muscles aren't fatigued by the third set, she needs to up the weight.

ATTITUDE

Staying positive is key to any weight-loss plan, says Dr. Kearney-Cooke. If Lisa beats herself up emotionally for every bad choice, it can set her on a negative spiral. Here's how to stay on track.

Don't dwell on a misstep. Forgive yourself, then just choose better the next time. And each day, jot down the healthy choices you made. Acknowledging the good helps boost self-esteem.

Her Results

Lost 10 pounds and ½ inch off waist

"This experience opened my eyes. I am much more conscious of my portions, and I walk instead of taking the subway whenever possible. The reason I've struggled with my weight, though, is my attitude: I get upset if I put on a few pounds, and go back to my bad habits. But I've learned if I 'screw up,' I can start fresh right away. That helped me focus on my program instead of trying to beat the scale. I wanted to lose 20 pounds; I lost half that, and I can still honestly say I'm proud of myself."

WARM UP TO WINTER WALKING

Even in the middle of winter, you can escape the treadmill and get outside! Our cold-weather picks will keep you safe and comfortable, whatever the weather.

LIGHT UP THE NIGHT. Tiny reflectors woven into illumiNITE's Cresta Microfleece Headband shine when a car's headlights hit them from up to 1,000 feet away. ($20, illuminite.com)

DON'T SLIP. The thin steel coils of the Yaktrax Pro grip snow and ice so you stay steady on slick ground. Just slide a pair over your usual walking shoes and go! ($30, yaktrax.com)

STAY DRY. The waterproof Keen Betty Boot shuts out slush like a snow boot but is flexible and lightweight enough to double as a walking shoe. Inside, bamboo-based insulation wicks moisture if you work up a sweat. ($120, www.keenfootwear.com)

KEEP WARM. Chilly spring walks call for layers that can be peeled off as you heat up. Skip jacket wrangling and try arm warmers instead. A favorite of ballerinas and cyclists, they're now popular on the walking circuit because they slip off as easily as gloves, without slowing you down. (EMS.com $20–$30, pearlizumi.com)

BANISH FROZEN FINGERTIPS. Wind-resistant 180s Puffy Quilt Gloves have a microfleece lining that traps heat. Bonus: Special finger pads allow you to adjust your iPod volume without baring your hands. ($40, www.palmflex.com)

INSULATE COLD TOES. Drymax Cold Weather Running Socks protect the tops of your feet (where wind hits first) with three ultrawarm layers, while hollow fibers throughout insulate and capture body heat. Plus, Drymax technology repels dampness, keeping feet cozy. ($15, drymaxsocks.com)

Bonus Weight-Loss
COOKBOOK

The recipes on the following pages show how you can eat well and still lose weight. Fight fat with delicious dishes such as Berry Good Peanut Butter Scones, Vegetable Chili, Cinnamon Sweet Potatoes with Vanilla, Orange-Glazed Ham, and Pumpkin Pecan Pie.

30 DELICIOUS RECIPES

BREAKFASTS

APPETIZERS

SALADS AND SOUPS

SIDES

MAIN DISHES

DESSERTS

MORE-VEGETABLE-THAN-EGG FRITTATA

MAKES 4 SERVINGS

For vegetables, try asparagus, mushrooms, zucchini, spinach, or Swiss chard. A frittata is a great way to use cooked vegetables, too. Instead of 4 cups raw veggies, add about 2 cups cooked to the onions, give a couple of good stirs, and proceed to step two.

2 tablespoons olive oil

½ onion, sliced

4 cups mixed vegetables (we used sliced Swiss chard, cut-up asparagus, and diced zucchini)

1 teaspoon salt

¼ cup fresh basil leaves (optional)

3 large eggs

½ cup freshly grated Parmesan cheese (optional)

Freshly ground black pepper

1. **PUT** 1 tablespoon of the oil in a 12" nonstick, ovenproof skillet over medium heat. When hot, add the onion and cook for 3 minutes, or until soft. Add the vegetables and ¼ teaspoon of the salt. Raise the heat to medium-high and cook, stirring occasionally, for 10 minutes, or until softened. Adjust the heat as necessary so the vegetables brown a little without scorching.

2. **TURN** the heat to low when the vegetables are nearly done and add the basil, if desired. Cook, stirring occasionally for up to 5 minutes longer, or until the pan is almost dry.

3. **BEAT** the eggs and cheese, if desired, in a bowl while the vegetables cook. Season with the remaining ¾ teaspoon salt and pepper. Add the remaining 1 tablespoon oil to the pan. Pour in the eggs, using a spoon if necessary to distribute them evenly. Cook, undisturbed, for 10 minutes, or until the eggs are barely set. Run under the broiler for a minute or two to brown very slightly.

4. **CUT** the frittata into wedges and serve hot, warm, or at room temperature.

PER SERVING: 136 calories, 7 g protein, 5 g carbohydrates, 2 g fiber, 10.5 g fat (2 g saturated), 665 mg sodium

CHOCOLATE-STUFFED FRENCH TOAST

MAKES 4 SERVINGS

Could there be anything better than chocolate for breakfast? Look to this dish when you want a decadent start to your weekend. Neufchâtel cheese contains one-third less fat than regular cream cheese, making it a great alternative in most recipes.

4 ounces semisweet chocolate, finely chopped

3 ounces Neufchâtel cheese, at room temperature

2 cups sliced strawberries

1 tablespoon sugar

1 teaspoon grated orange zest

6 ounces Italian bread, cut on the diagonal into 8 slices (½" thick)

2 large eggs

2 large egg whites

1 teaspoon vanilla extract

1 tablespoon trans-free margarine

1. **COMBINE** the chocolate and cheese in a small bowl and mix well. Combine the strawberries, sugar, and orange zest in a separate bowl.

2. **SPREAD** one-fourth of the chocolate mixture on 4 slices of the bread. Top each with a second slice and press lightly to form a sandwich.

3. **COMBINE** the whole eggs, egg whites, and vanilla extract in a medium bowl. Working one a time, dip both sides of each sandwich in the egg mixture and set on a plate.

4. **MELT** the margarine in a large nonstick skillet over medium heat. Wait for the foam to subside, then add the sandwiches and cook for 4 minutes per side, or until golden and cooked through. Serve hot, topped with the strawberry mixture.

PER SERVING: 410 calories, 14 g protein, 48 g carbohydrates, 5 g fiber, 20 g fat (10 g saturated), 420 mg sodium

WALNUT-PEAR PANCAKE WITH MAPLE SYRUP

MAKES 6 SERVINGS

Also known as a Dutch baby, this German-style baked pancake is a real crowd-pleaser. Once out of the oven, it deflates quickly, but it stays delicious to the last bite.

2 tablespoons trans-free margarine

2 pears, peeled, cored, and sliced

5 tablespoons sugar

1 cup all-purpose flour

¼ teaspoon ground cinnamon

¼ teaspoon salt

1 cup 1% milk

3 large eggs, lightly beaten

1½ teaspoons vanilla extract

1¼ cups walnuts, chopped

¼ cup maple syrup

1. PREHEAT the oven to 400°F.

2. MELT the margarine in a large ovenproof nonstick skillet over medium-high heat. Add the pears and cook, stirring occasionally, for 4 to 5 minutes, or until lightly browned and tender. Stir in 2 tablespoons of the sugar and cook for 1 minute longer. Remove from the heat.

3. MEANWHILE, combine the flour, cinnamon, salt, and the remaining 3 tablespoons sugar in a bowl. Stir in the milk, eggs, and vanilla extract until smooth. Fold in the walnuts.

4. POUR the batter over the pears and transfer the skillet to the oven. Bake for 22 to 24 minutes, or until the pancake is puffed and golden. Cut into 6 wedges. Drizzle with the maple syrup and serve hot.

PER SERVING: 395 calories, 10 g protein, 49 g carbohydrates, 4 g fiber, 19 g fat (2.5 g saturated), 180 mg sodium

BERRY GOOD PEANUT BUTTER SCONES

MAKES 8 SCONES

Because of the berry mixture they contain, these grab-and-go scones actually taste remarkably like peanut butter and jelly sandwiches—but with far less mess!

2 cups all-purpose flour

½ cup packed light brown sugar

1 teaspoon baking soda

1 teaspoon cream of tartar

¼ teaspoon salt

1 cup natural unsalted creamy peanut butter

1 package (5 ounces) mixed dried berries (about 1 cup)

¾ cup fat-free plain Greek yogurt

1 large egg

1. **PREHEAT** the oven to 400°F. Line a heavy baking sheet with parchment paper.

2. **COMBINE** the flour, brown sugar, baking soda, cream of tartar, and salt in a food processor. Pulse to combine.

3. **ADD** the peanut butter by spoonfuls to the flour mixture. Pulse until the mixture is combined and looks like sand. Transfer to a mixing bowl and stir in the berries.

4. **STIR** the yogurt and egg together in a small bowl and add to the flour mixture. Stir with a spoon until combined. Use your hands, if necessary, to ensure that all the flour is incorporated.

5. **TRANSFER** the dough to a lightly floured work surface and pat into a circle about 1" thick. Cut the dough into 8 equal wedges. Arrange the wedges on the baking sheet and bake for 15 minutes, or until lightly browned. Let cool slightly and serve warm.

PER SERVING: 429 calories, 13 g protein, 58 g carbohydrates, 4 g fiber, 17 g fat (2 g saturated), 250 mg sodium

LEMON-BLUEBERRY BUTTERMILK MUFFINS

MAKES 6 SERVINGS

Lemons and blueberries are a perfect combination, and this recipe affords you two muffins as a serving! What could be better than that?

1¾ cups cake flour

⅔ cup blueberries

⅔ cup sugar

¾ cup low-fat buttermilk

6 tablespoons canola oil

2 large eggs

1 tablespoon grated lemon zest

¾ teaspoon lemon extract

1½ teaspoons baking powder

¼ teaspoon baking soda

¼ teaspoon salt

1. **PREHEAT** the oven to 375°F. Line a 12-cup muffin pan with paper liners. Measure out 2 tablespoons of the flour in a small bowl. Add the blueberries and toss. Set aside.

2. **COMBINE** the sugar, buttermilk, oil, eggs, and lemon zest and extract in a large bowl. Combine the remaining flour, the baking powder, baking soda, and salt in a separate bowl. Add the flour mixture to the buttermilk mixture and stir until smooth. (The batter will be thin.) Fold in the reserved blueberries.

3. **FILL** the muffin cups two-thirds full and bake for 16 to 17 minutes, or until the tops are lightly golden and a toothpick inserted in the center comes out clean. Cool in the pan on a rack for 5 minutes. Remove the muffins from the pan and cool completely on the rack.

PER SERVING: 402 calories, 7 g protein, 58 g carbohydrates, 1 g fiber, 16 g fat (2 g saturated), 330 mg sodium

MANGO-AVOCADO SALSA

MAKES 4 SERVINGS

Mango and pineapple lends a sunny look, as well as lots of flavor, to this delicious salsa. If your family prefers a little spice, a few splashes of hot sauce will do the trick.

1 mango

1 Hass avocado

⅓ fresh pineapple

¼ red onion

2 tablespoons chopped fresh cilantro

1 tablespoon fresh lime juice

¼ teaspoon salt

4 ounces baked tortilla chips

1. CHOP the mango into ¼" to ½" pieces. Chop the avocado into ½" cubes. Chop the pineapple into ¼" to ½" pieces. Finely chop the onion.

2. COMBINE the mango, avocado, pineapple, onion, cilantro, lime juice, and salt in a bowl. Serve with the tortilla chips.

PER SERVING: 265 calories, 10 g protein, 44 g carbohydrates, 6 g fiber, 10 g fat (1.5 g saturated), 430 mg sodium

ASIAN SNACK MIX

MAKES 10 SERVINGS

This snack mix can have a "wild" side if you make it with wasabi-coated peanuts. Just add 2½ cups wasabi-coated peanuts in place of the regular peanuts after the snack mix bakes.

2 tablespoons canola oil

2 teaspoons reduced-sodium soy sauce

¼ teaspoon garlic powder

¼ teaspoon ground ginger

2 cups toasted rice cereal squares

2 cups air-popped popcorn

1¼ cups unsalted dry-roasted peanuts

1. PREHEAT the oven to 325°F. Coat a large rimmed baking sheet with cooking spray.

2. WHISK together the oil, soy sauce, garlic powder, and ginger in a large bowl. Add the cereal, popcorn, and peanuts, tossing to coat evenly. Spread the mixture on the baking sheet. Bake for 15 minutes, stirring occasionally, until the cereal is very crisp. Watch carefully so the mixture does not burn.

3. REMOVE from the oven and let cool completely before storing in an airtight container.

PER SERVING: 180 calories, 5 g protein, 10 g carbohydrates, 2 g fiber, 15 g fat (1.5 g saturated), 80 mg sodium

TOMATO AND ROASTED PEPPER BRUSCHETTA

MAKES 4 SERVINGS

How can you tell when a tomato is perfectly ripe? Your nose knows. A ripe tomato smells like a tomato; unripe ones have no aroma.

2 small baguettes (about 4 ounces each), cut on the diagonal into 16 slices total

¼ cup extra-virgin olive oil

1 small clove garlic

1 tomato, seeded and chopped

1 roasted pepper, patted dry and chopped (about ½ cup)

½ small red onion, finely chopped

2 tablespoons chopped fresh basil

1 tablespoon balsamic vinegar

⅛ teaspoon salt

¼ teaspoon ground black pepper

1. PREHEAT the oven to 400°F.

2. ARRANGE the baguette slices on a baking sheet in a single layer. Brush the tops with 2 tablespoons of the oil and bake for 7 to 8 minutes, or until crisp. Remove from the oven, let cool 1 minute, then rub the top of each slice with the garlic clove.

3. MEANWHILE, combine the remaining 2 tablespoons oil, the tomato, roasted pepper, onion, basil, vinegar, salt, and black pepper in a bowl. Spoon the mixture over the slices of toast and serve.

PER SERVING: 329 calories, 8 g protein, 40 g carbohydrates, 2 g fiber, 15 g fat (2.5 g saturated), 570 mg sodium

EASY BARBECUE PITA PIZZAS

MAKES 2 SERVINGS

When you need a pizza fix, this recipe will do the trick, especially if you love thin crusts. Adding a layer of olive oil between the pita and the sauce helps make the bread extra crispy.

2 whole wheat pitas (6"), split horizontally in half

2 tablespoons olive oil

4 tablespoons barbecue sauce

½ cup (2 ounces) shredded reduced-fat Cheddar cheese

4 ounces cooked chicken breast, sliced

2 scallions, thinly sliced

Chili powder (optional)

1. PREHEAT the oven to 375°F.

2. ARRANGE the pita halves rough side up on a baking sheet and drizzle 1½ teaspoons of the oil on each. Use the back of a spoon to spread the oil evenly to the edges. Top each with 1 tablespoon barbecue sauce, 2 tablespoons cheese, ¼ of the chicken, and ¼ of the scallions. Sprinkle with chili powder, if desired. Bake for 7 minutes, or until the cheese is melted.

PER SERVING: 410 calories, 24 g protein, 39 g carbohydrates, 4 g fiber, 18 g fat (3.5 g saturated), 730 mg sodium

PISTACHIO CHEESE SPREAD

MAKES 4 SERVINGS

Greek feta cheese adds tang to this spread. For a slightly less assertive spread, replace 1 ounce of the feta with 1 ounce fat-free cream cheese; the calories will be only slightly lower (273).

½ cup shelled unsalted roasted pistachios

2 ounces reduced-fat feta cheese, at room temperature

2 ounces fat-free cream cheese, at room temperature

1 tablespoon honey

1 tablespoon water

1 teaspoon salt-free lemon-pepper seasoning

2 whole grain pitas (6")

1. PLACE the pistachios in a food processor and pulse 6 to 8 times to chop coarsely. Add the feta, cream cheese, honey, water, and lemon-pepper seasoning. Pulse to incorporate.

2. SPLIT the pitas horizontally in half and toast to desired crispness. Cut each pita into 8 wedges for a total of 32 and serve with the spread.

PER SERVING: 280 calories, 13 g protein, 26 g carbohydrates, 5 g fiber, 16 g fat (3 g saturated), 400 mg sodium

TOMATO-OLIVE SALAD

MAKES 4 SERVINGS

Fennel is the secret ingredient in this summery salad. Look for it near the leafy greens in your grocery's produce section. For extra flavor, chop some of the delicate, dill-like fronds and toss them into the salad, too.

4 cups shredded romaine

2 cups grape tomatoes, halved

1 cucumber, halved lengthwise and thinly sliced crosswise

20 pitted large black olives, sliced

20 pitted kalamata olives, sliced

½ fennel bulb, thinly sliced

½ small red onion, thinly sliced

2 tablespoons extra-virgin olive oil

4 teaspoons balsamic vinegar

¼ teaspoon salt

¼ teaspoon ground black pepper

1. **COMBINE** the romaine, tomatoes, cucumber, olives, fennel, and onion in a large bowl.

2. **ADD** the oil, vinegar, salt, and black pepper and toss well.

PER SERVING: 184 calories, 2 g protein, 12 g carbohydrates, 4 g fiber, 15 g fat (2 g saturated), 670 mg sodium

ROASTED BEET SALAD

MAKES 4 SERVINGS

The addition of lightly cooked pears to this classic salad combination will likely make this already sweet vegetable more palatable to even the most picky eaters.

4 medium beets (about 1½ pounds), ends trimmed

½ cup balsamic vinegar

2 tablespoons sugar

½ cup walnuts, coarsely chopped

2 teaspoons olive oil

2 pears, peeled, cored, and cut into 8 wedges each

½ teaspoon salt

¼ teaspoon ground black pepper

2 cups arugula (optional)

4 tablespoons (1 ounce) crumbled blue cheese

1. **PREHEAT** the oven to 425°F.

2. **WRAP** the beets in foil and set on a baking sheet. Bake for 1 hour, or until a knife easily pierces the beets. Remove from the oven and let cool for 30 minutes. Peel the beets, cut each into 8 wedges (wear disposable rubber gloves if you're concerned about the beets staining your hands), and transfer to a bowl.

3. **MEANWHILE,** combine the vinegar and sugar in a small saucepan. Bring the mixture to a boil over medium-high heat and cook for 5 to 6 minutes, or until reduced by about half and thick enough to coat the back of a spoon. Set aside.

4. **PLACE** the walnuts in a large nonstick skillet and cook over medium-high heat, shaking the pan often, for 2 to 3 minutes, or until lightly toasted. Transfer to the bowl with the beets.

5. **ADD** the oil to the skillet and return to medium-high heat. Add the pears and cook for 2 minutes per side, or until lightly browned. Remove from the heat. Add the reserved vinegar mixture, salt, and pepper to the beets, tossing to coat well. Place ½ cup arugula, if desired, on each of 4 plates and top with the beet mixture and pears. Sprinkle each serving with 1 table-spoon blue cheese.

PER SERVING: 301 calories, 7 g protein, 42 g carbohydrates, 8 g fiber, 13 g fat (2.5 g saturated), 550 mg sodium

GREEN BEAN AND PUMPKIN SEED SALAD

MAKES 4 SERVINGS

The contrast between the tender beans and crunchy pumpkin seeds makes this salad especially appealing. Serve with grilled pork tenderloin.

¼ cup water

2 teaspoons canola oil

½ teaspoon ground cumin

⅛ teaspoon salt

¾ pound green beans, broken into 2" lengths (about 3 cups)

½ cup shelled unsalted dry-roasted pumpkin seeds

½ small red onion, halved and thinly sliced

1 tablespoon fresh lime juice

1. **COMBINE** the water, oil, cumin, and salt in a large nonstick skillet. Cover and bring to a boil over high heat. Reduce the heat to medium. Add the beans and stir. Cook, tossing occasionally, for 5 minutes, or until the beans are tender and all the water is gone.

2. **ADD** the pumpkin seeds and cook, tossing, for about 2 minutes, or until the seeds are hot.

3. **TRANSFER** the mixture to a serving platter. Add the onion and lime juice and toss to combine.

PER SERVING: 140 calories, 5 g protein, 9 g carbohydrates, 3 g fiber, 10 g fat (1.5 g saturated), 75 mg sodium

VEGETABLE CHILI

MAKES 6 SERVINGS

Kidney beans or pinto beans are a traditional starting point, but if you want to get creative, try chickpeas, black beans, cannellini beans, navy beans, or even lentils.

3 tablespoons olive oil

½ pound ground beef, pork, turkey, or chicken (optional)

1 onion, finely chopped

3 cloves garlic, minced

1 or 2 small eggplant, cubed

1 medium zucchini, chopped (or use more eggplant)

2 carrots, chopped

1 cup quartered mushrooms

¼ teaspoons crushed red-pepper flakes

4 cups canned kidney or pinto beans, rinsed and drained

1 box (26 ounces) chopped tomatoes (about 3 cups) (we used Pomi)

1¾ teaspoons salt

1 teaspoon ground cumin

1 teaspoon dried oregano

4 cups water or broth

½ teaspoon freshly ground black pepper

2 tablespoons chopped fresh cilantro or parsley (optional)

1. **HEAT** the oil in a large Dutch oven over medium heat. When hot, add the meat. Season with salt and cook, stirring frequently, for 5 minutes, or until well-browned all over. Remove the meat from the pan and drain off all but 3 tablespoons of the fat. (If you're skipping the meat, put some oil in the pan and start the recipe here.)

2. **RETURN** the Dutch oven to the stove over medium-high heat. Add the onion and garlic. Cook and stir for 1 minute, or until just softened. Add the eggplant, zucchini, carrots, mushrooms, and red-pepper flakes. Cook, stirring occasionally, for 15 to 20 minutes, or until the vegetables begin to soften, adjusting the heat so that nothing scorches.

3. **ADD** the beans, tomatoes (with juice), salt, cumin, and oregano. Return the meat to the Dutch oven. Add enough water to submerge everything. Bring the mixture to a boil, reduce the heat to medium, and cook, stirring occasionally and adding more liquid if necessary, for 15 minutes. Add the black pepper, season with more salt to taste, and sprinkle with the cilantro or parsley, if desired.

PER SERVING: 266 calories, 12 g protein, 37 g carbohydrates, 13 g fiber, 8 g fat (1 g saturated), 943 mg sodium

LENTIL AND BEAN SOUP

MAKES 4 SERVINGS

Make it your way! To add meat, brown a pound of ground pork with the onion, and use 1 cup of lentils and 4 cups of water. Vegans can replace the smoked cheese with diced, dried spiced tofu. This easy, inexpensive recipe will save you time and money. It's even better reheated. You can prepare the soup up to the final step up to a week before serving. The flavors will develop. If it gets too thick, just add enough water to make it soupy again.

1 onion, chopped

1 tablespoon olive oil

2 teaspoons chili powder

½ teaspoon salt

1¼ cups dried lentils

5 cups water

1 can (8 ounces) tomato sauce

3 carrots, chopped

3 ribs celery, chopped

1 can (15½ ounces) great Northern or black beans, rinsed and drained

3½ ounces smoked Gouda, shredded

2 tablespoons fresh cilantro, parsley, and/or scallion tops, chopped, or 1½ teaspoons freeze-dried chives

Salt

Freshly ground black pepper

¼ cup sour cream (optional)

1. **SAUTÉ** the onion in the oil in a Dutch oven over medium-high heat for 5 minutes, until golden. Stir in the chili powder and salt.

2. **ADD** the lentils and water. Bring to a boil. Reduce the heat to medium and simmer for 5 minutes. Add the tomato sauce, carrots, and celery. Simmer for 10 minutes. Add the beans and cook for 5 minutes, or until the vegetables are tender.

3. **STIR** in the cheese and herbs. Season to taste with salt and black pepper. Serve topped with the sour cream, if desired.

PER SERVING: 480 calories, 30 g protein, 68 g carbohydrates, 21 g fiber, 12 g fat (5 g saturated), 869 mg sodium

SIDES

CINNAMON SWEET POTATOES WITH VANILLA

MAKES 8 SERVINGS

Smart splurge: Just a tablespoon of butter makes these potatoes taste luscious. You can make these up to 5 days ahead, and they reheat beautifully. If they're a bit dry, just stir in water.

3 pounds sweet potatoes, peeled and cut into approximately 3" chunks

1 cup reduced-sodium chicken broth

½ teaspoon ground cinnamon

⅔ cup fat-free milk "plus" (we used Over the Moon)

1 tablespoon butter

1 teaspoon vanilla extract

Salt

Freshly ground black pepper

1. PLACE the potatoes and broth in a large pot with a tight-fitting lid and bring to a simmer over medium heat. Cook for 25 minutes, or until the potatoes are fork-tender.

2. ADD the cinnamon, milk, and butter.

3. MASH in a food processor or with a handheld masher until smooth. Add the vanilla extract and season with salt and black pepper to taste.

PER SERVING: 125 calories, 3 g protein, 25 g carbohydrates, 3 g fiber, 2 g fat (1 g saturated), 126 mg sodium

WHOLE GRAIN STUFFING WITH SAUSAGE

MAKES 8 SERVINGS

Whole wheat bread and smoked turkey sausage add healthy flavor in this moist-on-the-inside, crisp-on-top dressing. You can put this stuffing together a few days before serving or up to 2 weeks ahead, then freeze it. Cover and store; thaw when ready to bake.

2 teaspoons canola oil

1 large onion, chopped

½ teaspoon salt

3 large ribs celery, chopped (about 2 cups)

3 tablespoons thinly sliced fresh sage leaves or 1 tablespoon dried

2 cloves garlic, minced or crushed

1½ teaspoons whole fennel seeds (optional)

1½ cups fat-free milk "plus" (we used Over the Moon)

½ cup reduced-sodium chicken broth

1 sliced bakery loaf 100% whole wheat bread (about 1 pound), cut into bite-size cubes (about 10 cups)

8 ounces cooked smoked turkey or chicken sausage, chopped

Salt

Freshly ground black pepper

1. **PREHEAT** the oven to 350°F. Lightly coat an 11" x 7" baking dish with oil or cooking spray.

2. **PUT** the canola oil in the Dutch oven over medium heat. Add the onion and salt and cook, stirring occasionally, for 25 minutes, or until the onion turns golden.

3. **ADD** the celery, sage, garlic, and fennel seeds, if desired, and cook for 5 minutes.

4. **REMOVE** from the heat and add the milk, broth, bread, and sausage. Stir well, season to taste with salt and pepper, and put in the prepared baking dish.

5. **COAT** the top of the stuffing lightly with more oil or cooking spray, cover the dish with foil, and bake for 30 minutes. Remove the foil and continue to bake for 40 minutes, or until the top is brown and crisp.

PER SERVING: 243 calories, 11 g protein, 35 g carbohydrates, 4 g fiber, 7 g fat (1.5 g saturated), 619 mg sodium

ROASTED CAULIFLOWER PARMESAN

MAKES 8 SERVINGS

This dish can be cooked while your main dish is baking or roasting, or you can make it 2 to 3 hours beforehand and heat it just before serving. If you don't have room in your oven for two pans, cook one at a time, then combine all the cauliflower on a single pan and reheat together briefly.

1 large head cauliflower (about 2 pounds), stemmed and cut into 1" to 3" slices

½ cup grated Parmesan cheese (about 1½ ounces)

Salt

Freshly ground black pepper

1. **PREHEAT** the oven to 350°F. Line 2 large rimmed baking sheets with foil or parchment paper and lightly coat or spray with oil.

2. **ARRANGE** the cauliflower on the pans without overlapping. Sprinkle with the cheese and bake on the top rack for 40 minutes, or until golden brown. Season with salt and pepper to taste.

PER SERVING: 47 calories, 4 g protein, 6 g carbohydrates, 3 g fiber, 1.5 g fat (1 g saturated), 116 mg sodium

BROILED ASPARAGUS

MAKES 8 SERVINGS

This is the perfect side dish for any meat. Trim the asparagus by washing it and bending each stem until it breaks naturally.

2 pounds asparagus, trimmed

3 tablespoons olive oil

Salt

1. **PREHEAT** the broiler. Put the rack in the middle position.

2. **PUT** the asparagus in a roasting pan. Toss with the oil to coat. Arrange the asparagus evenly in a single layer. Sprinkle with salt to taste.

3. **BROIL** the asparagus for 5 minutes, or until nearly done. Shake the pan to turn the spears and broil about 3 minutes longer.

PER SERVING: 57 calories, 1 g protein, 2 g carbohydrates, 1 g fiber, 5 g fat (0.5 g saturated), 1 mg sodium

CREAMY CARAMELIZED ONIONS AND CARROTS

MAKES 8 SERVINGS

Our creamed onions taste sweet, thanks to caramelizing them and adding carrots. You can make this vegetable dish hours or even days before serving. If the sauce is too thick when reheated, just stir in water bit by bit until it's the consistency you want.

1 tablespoon butter

2 large onions, thinly sliced

¾ teaspoon salt

1½ teaspoons ground coriander seed (optional)

3 pounds carrots, cut into ¼" slices

1½ cups fat-free milk "plus" (we used Over the Moon)

1 tablespoon cornstarch

Salt

Freshly ground black pepper

1 tablespoon finely chopped fresh chives (optional)

1. MELT the butter in a large, heavy-bottom pot with a lid over medium-low heat. Add the onion and salt and cook, stirring occasionally, for 50 minutes, or until the onion browns.

2. STIR in the coriander (if using). Add the carrots, cover, and cook over medium heat for 20 minutes, or until just tender.

3. WHISK the milk and cornstarch together until dissolved. Stir into the carrot mixture.

4. HEAT until the liquid comes to a simmer. Season with salt and pepper to taste. Serve sprinkled with the chives, if desired.

PER SERVING: 111 calories, 3 g protein, 21 g carbohydrates, 5 g fiber, 2 g fat (1 g saturated), 359 mg sodium

MAIN DISHES

GINGERED CHICKEN AND GREENS STIR-FRY

MAKES 4 SERVINGS

This is an ideal way to use leftover greens. If you're cooking them fresh, sauté them in the same pan you'll use to stir-fry for easy cleanup.

1 tablespoon canola oil

1 tablespoon finely chopped fresh ginger

2 cloves garlic, thinly sliced

6 scallions, thinly sliced (keep bulbs and leaves separate)

1 large red bell pepper, cut into thin strips

1 pound boneless, skinless chicken thighs, cut into ½" strips

¼ teaspoon salt

2 cups cooked greens, about 1 pound raw with stems (we used mustard greens)

1 tablespoon soy sauce

2 teaspoons toasted sesame oil

1. **PUT** the canola oil in a large stainless steel or nonstick frying pan or wok over medium-high heat. When hot, add the ginger, garlic, and scallion bulbs. Stir-fry for 2 minutes.

2. **ADD** the pepper and stir-fry for 2 minutes. Add the chicken and salt and stir-fry for 5 minutes, or until almost done.

3. **STIR** in the cooked greens, scallion leaves, soy sauce, and sesame oil. Add more salt to taste.

PER SERVING: 289 calories, 22 g protein, 9 g carbohydrates, 3 g fiber, 18.5 g fat (4 g saturated), 623 mg sodium

TRADITIONAL PAELLA

MAKES 6 SERVINGS

Don't be troubled if your paella forms a crust on the bottom as it cooks. Paella aficionados consider these chewy bits the best part! Be sure to dislodge it with a spatula so everyone can have a taste. Variation: Skinned chicken drumsticks can stand in for thighs.

3 tablespoons olive oil

6 boneless, skinless chicken thighs (about 1¼ pounds)

½ pound fresh turkey or chicken sausages or chorizo

1 green bell pepper, chopped

½ red onion, chopped

2 cloves garlic, minced

1½ teaspoons paprika

1 teaspoon dried oregano

1 teaspoon dried thyme

¼ teaspoon freshly ground black pepper

⅛ teaspoon ground red pepper

1½ cups short- or long-grain rice

2⅔ cups chicken broth (we used Kitchen Basics)

¾ teaspoon salt

1 pound peeled shrimp

1 cup frozen peas

¼ cup chopped fresh parsley

1. **HEAT** the oil in a paella pan or Dutch oven over medium heat. Sprinkle the chicken with salt and pepper and add it and the sausages to the pan. Cook, turning, for 10 minutes, or until the sausages are browned and almost cooked through. Remove the chicken and sausages.

2. **ADD** the bell pepper and onion, sprinkle with salt, and cook for 5 minutes, or until softened. Stir in the garlic, paprika, oregano, thyme, and black and red peppers and cook for 1 minute. Add the rice and then the broth and salt. Bring to a boil, return the chicken to the pan, reduce the heat to low, cover, and cook for 15 minutes.

3. **SLICE** the sausages and stir into the paella along with the shrimp, peas, and 2 tablespoons of the parsley. Season to taste with salt and pepper. Cover and cook 5 minutes longer. Remove from the heat and let stand, covered, for 5 minutes. Serve sprinkled with the remaining 2 tablespoons parsley.

PER SERVING: 555 calories, 50 g protein, 50 g carbohydrates, 3 g fiber, 16 g fat (3.5 g saturated), 904 mg sodium

TOMATO-TOPPED MEAT LOAF

Use your favorite Italian seasoning—rosemary, oregano, basil, thyme, parsley, or a combination—in these beefy, juicy, yet low-fat individual meat loaves. Here's how to cut onions without tears: Work near a kitchen exhaust fan or don glasses (even sunglasses!). Using onions right from the fridge, rather than at room temperature, helps, too.

1 pound 90% lean ground beef

1 medium onion, minced or grated

½ cup dried bread crumbs

3 tablespoons 1% milk

1 large egg

1 tablespoon coarse-ground or Dijon mustard

1 tablespoon finely chopped flat-leaf parsley (optional)

1½ teaspoons dried Italian herbs

1 teaspoon garlic powder

1 teaspoon salt

¾ teaspoon freshly ground black pepper

⅔ cup tomato basil pasta sauce

1. PREHEAT the oven to 425°F. Spray a baking sheet with oil.

2. MIX the beef, onion, crumbs, milk, egg, mustard, parsley (if desired), herbs, garlic powder, salt, black pepper, and half of the pasta sauce until the ingredients are evenly distributed.

3. DIVIDE the mixture into quarters and put them on a prepared baking sheet. Form into loaf shapes and spoon the remaining pasta sauce over the top of each. Bake for 20 minutes, or until brown and cooked through.

PER SERVING: 280 calories, 26 g protein, 18 g carbohydrates, 1 g fiber, 11.5 g fat (4.5 g saturated), 925 mg sodium

ORANGE-GLAZED HAM

MAKES 8 SERVINGS PLUS GENEROUS LEFTOVERS

This is a real crowd-pleaser. If you have a larger ham, just multiply the glaze. For a 15-pounder, double the glaze and bake the ham for 3 hours, glazing after 2. You can't go wrong, as long as the ham is heated through and the top is dark and crisp.

7 pound bone-in ham

16 whole cloves

¼ cup orange marmalade

¼ cup brown sugar

3 tablespoons Dijon mustard

1. **PREHEAT** the oven to 350°F.

2. **PUT** the ham in a roasting pan, fat side up. Score 16 diamonds on the fat side of the ham and put a clove in the center of each one.

3. **BAKE** on the bottom rack of the oven for 1 hour.

4. **MIX** the marmalade, sugar, and mustard together in a bowl. Remove the ham from the oven and coat with the glaze.

5. **COOK** the ham for 1 hour longer, or until the internal temperature reaches 140°F, glazing it twice.

6. **REMOVE** the ham from the oven and let stand for 30 minutes.

PER 4-OUNCE SERVING: 174 calories, 30 g protein, 7 g carbohydrates, 0 g fiber, 3.5 g fat (1 g saturated), 999 mg sodium

COD CAKES

MAKES 4 SERVINGS

Try these crisp and delicious patties with any fish you like. You can also use canned or leftover fish, instead of starting from scratch. Just substitute two large cans of salmon or tuna, drained, or 2 cups of flaked cooked fish for the cod.

1 pound cod, cut into large chunks

½ teaspoon salt

¼ cup + 2 tablespoons 2% Greek yogurt

¼ cup chopped fresh parsley

1 egg yolk, beaten

1 tablespoon Dijon mustard

1 tablespoon freshly squeezed lemon juice (from ½ lemon)

¾ cup + 2 tablespoons panko (we used Progresso) or bread crumbs

3 scallions, minced

¼ teaspoon freshly ground black pepper

¼ cup canola oil

1. **STEAM** the fish: Put about an inch of water in the bottom of a large nonstick skillet and bring to a simmer over medium-high heat. Season the fish with ¼ teaspoon of the salt and add it to the pan. Cover the pan and simmer the fish over low heat for 6 to 8 minutes, or until just done. Remove from the pan with a slotted spoon and drain on paper towels. Pour out the water and dry the pan. Allow the fish to cool slightly, about 5 minutes, and pat completely dry.

2. **FLAKE** the fish in a medium bowl with forks or your fingers, removing any bones as you go. Add the yogurt, parsley, egg yolk, mustard, lemon juice, 6 tablespoons of the panko, the scallions, pepper, and the remaining ¼ teaspoon salt. Stir to combine.

3. **SHAPE** the mixture into eight round cakes. Coat the cakes with the remaining ½ cup panko and pat off the excess.

4. **HEAT** 2 tablespoons of the oil in the nonstick skillet over medium heat. Add the cakes and cook for 2 to 3 minutes, or until brown and crisp. Add the remaining 2 tablespoons oil, turn the cakes, and cook for 2 to 3 minutes longer, or until golden brown on the other side. Drain on paper towels. Serve hot with your choice of dipping sauce.

PER SERVING: 291 calories, 22 g protein, 12 g carbohydrates, 1 g fiber, 16.5 g fat (2 g saturated), 492 mg sodium

DESSERTS

PUMPKIN PECAN PIE

MAKES 8 SERVINGS

This recipe combines traditional holiday flavors into one spectacular dessert. The gingersnap crust alone saves 5 grams of saturated fat per slice over a traditional pie with made-from-scratch pastry dough. Just the right amount of nutritious pecans creates the delicious—and beautiful—topping without sending calories through the roof.

¼ cup butter

1¼ cups gingersnap cookie crumbs (about 30 cookies)

1½ teaspoons vanilla extract

1 can (15 ounces) pure pumpkin

1 large egg

1 large egg white

½ teaspoon ground cinnamon

¼ teaspoon ground nutmeg

¾ cup dark brown sugar

2 tablespoons honey

¾ cup pecan halves

1. **PREHEAT** the oven to 350°F.

2. **MELT** 2 tablespoons of the butter in the microwave and mix with the cookie crumbs and vanilla extract in a bowl. Press onto the bottom and sides of an 8" pie plate. Bake for 10 minutes and cool.

3. **BLEND** the pumpkin, egg, egg white, cinnamon, nutmeg, and ½ cup of the sugar. Spread in the crust.

4. **BAKE** for 35 to 40 minutes, or until the filling is set around the edges or a knife inserted in the center comes out clean.

5. **HEAT** the broiler. Combine the honey and the remaining ¼ cup sugar and 2 tablespoons butter in a small nonstick saucepan. Cook over low heat until the sugar dissolves, stirring constantly. Stir in the pecans to coat.

6. **SPREAD** the topping over the pie. Broil for 2 minutes, or until bubbly and golden brown (do not burn).

PER SERVING: 357 calories, 4 g protein, 51 g carbohydrates, 3 g fiber, 16.5 g fat (5 g saturated), 237 mg sodium

CHOCOLATE CUPCAKES WITH WHIPPED CREAM FROSTING

MAKES 8 SERVINGS

These cupcakes are rich and moist, without any butter. A big swirl of creamy vanilla frosting tastes heavenly, yet saves on calories and saturated fat compared with a typical buttercream frosting.

1¼ cups all-purpose flour

¾ cup granulated sugar

¼ cup unsweetened cocoa powder

1 teaspoon baking soda

⅛ teaspoon salt

½ cup water

½ cup fat-free plain yogurt

¼ cup vegetable oil

¼ cup unsweetened applesauce

1 large egg white

½ teaspoon instant coffee, dissolved in 2 tablespoons hot water

1½ teaspoons vanilla extract

½ cup + 2 tablespoons heavy cream

2 ounces reduced-fat cream cheese (Neufchâtel)

¼ cup confectioners' sugar

2–3 drops red food coloring (optional)

1. **PREHEAT** the oven to 350°F. Line 8 cups of a standard muffin tin or spray with oil.

2. **MIX** the flour, granulated sugar, cocoa, baking soda, and salt in a bowl with a fork.

3. **COMBINE** the water, yogurt, oil, applesauce, egg white, coffee, and 1 teaspoon of the vanilla extract in a large bowl. Beat with an electric mixer until combined and smooth. Slowly add the flour mixture and beat until smooth.

4. **FILL** the muffin cups with the batter. Bake for 20 to 25 minutes, or until a wooden pick inserted in the center of each cake comes out clean. Cool completely.

5. **BEAT** the cream, cream cheese, confectioners' sugar, and the remaining ½ teaspoon of vanilla extract in a bowl with an electric mixer until thick and stiff. Stir in the food coloring, if desired. Spread about 2 tablespoons of frosting on top of each cupcake. If not serving immediately, store the cupcakes in the refrigerator.

PER SERVING: 326 calories, 5 g protein, 42 g carbohydrates, 2 g fiber, 16.5 g fat (6.5 g saturated), 251 mg sodium

CHOCOLATE NO-BAKE CRUNCHIES

MAKES 3 DOZEN COOKIES

Crisp cornflakes and chewy raisins add a fun mix of textures as well as loads of flavor and nutrients to these mouthwatering dark chocolate confections.

½ cup semisweet chocolate chips

1 cup cornflakes

¼ cup raisins

1. **LINE** a baking sheet with wax paper.

2. **PUT** the chocolate chips in a medium microwaveable bowl. Microwave on high for 1 minute to melt. Stir until smooth. Gently fold the cereal and raisins into the chocolate until combined, being careful not to crush the cereal.

3. **DROP** the mixture by teaspoonfuls onto the prepared pan. Chill for 45 minutes.

PER COOKIE: 17 calories, 0 g protein, 3 g carbohydrates, 0 g fiber, 1 g fat (0.5 g saturated), 8 mg sodium

CHERRY-PISTACHIO BISCOTTI

MAKES 4½ DOZEN COOKIES

Studded with nuts and fruit, our biscotti are filling and scrumptious. They have 32 percent less saturated fat than the traditional cookie.

2 cups all-purpose flour

1 cup whole wheat flour

2 teaspoons baking powder

¼ teaspoon salt

1 cup sugar

¼ cup butter

2 tablespoons ⁵⁰⁄₅₀ butter blend spread (we used Smart Balance)

½ teaspoon almond extract

2 large eggs

⅔ cup pistachios, chopped

½ cup dried tart cherries or cherry-flavor sweetened dried cranberries

1. **PREHEAT** the oven to 350°F. Line a baking sheet with foil.

2. **WHISK** the flours, baking powder, and salt in a bowl.

3. **BEAT** the sugar, butter, spread, and almond extract in a medium bowl with an electric mixer on medium speed until combined. Beat in the eggs, one at a time. Beat in the dry ingredients in thirds. Add the pistachios and cherries and beat to combine.

4. **FORM** into 2 slightly flat 10" x 2½" logs. Put on the pan and bake for 35 minutes. Remove from the oven. Cover with a moist towel and let stand for 10 minutes. Cut crosswise into ⅓" slices. Lay cut side down on ungreased baking sheets. Bake for 12 minutes, turning once.

PER COOKIE: 66 calories, 1 g protein, 10 g carbohydrates, 1 g fiber, 2 g fat (1 g saturated), 29 mg sodium

PEPPERMINT SUGAR COOKIES

MAKES 2½ DOZEN COOKIES

Give cutout cookies extra flavor with festive peppermint. Top them with plain granulated sugar or have fun with colored sugars and candies. Sugar toppings are easier than icing, and they have at least 70 percent fewer calories than frosting—and no fat.

1¼ cups all-purpose flour

¼ cup whole wheat flour

⅛ teaspoon salt

½ cup sugar

¼ cup + 2 tablespoons butter

2 tablespoons ⁵⁰⁄₅₀ butter blend spread (we used Smart Balance)

1 large egg

¾ teaspoon peppermint extract

¼ cup sugar, colored sugar, sprinkles, or candy decorations

1. **WHISK** the flours and salt in a bowl.

2. **BEAT** the sugar, butter, and spread in a medium bowl with an electric mixer on medium speed until combined. Add the egg and peppermint extract and beat until combined. Add the dry ingredients in thirds, beating until smooth.

3. **ROLL** out half the dough between 2 pieces of plastic wrap until ¼" thick. Repeat with the remaining dough. Wrap in plastic wrap and chill for 30 minutes.

4. **PREHEAT** the oven to 350°F. Line 2 baking sheets with foil and lightly coat with cooking spray.

5. **REMOVE** the top sheet of plastic wrap and cut the cookies with 2" cookie cutters. Decorate with colored sugar or sprinkles. Peel the cookies from the bottom sheet of plastic and place 1½" apart on the prepared baking sheets. Reroll the scraps and repeat until all the dough is used, chilling as needed. Sprinkle with the sugar or press decorative candies lightly into the dough.

6. **BAKE** the cookies for 13 to 15 minutes, or until the edges are golden.

PER COOKIE: 72 calories, 1 g protein, 10 g carbohydrates, 0.5 g fiber, 3 g fat (2 g saturated), 13 mg sodium

BAKERS' SECRETS

FOR FASTER COOLING: Chill the dough for a little less than half the time in the freezer instead of the fridge.

FOR TIDY SHAPES: To keep the edges clean, make sure your cutter is free of dough, and dip it in flour after every few cookies. If the dough still sticks, chill it before continuing.

FOR LATER: The dough for almost any dropped, rolled, or shaped cookie can be formed into a log instead, wrapped well, and frozen. Double the recipe and put half away to bake later. When you're ready, just slice and bake.

"I WENT FROM SIZE 24 TO SIZE 6"

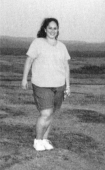

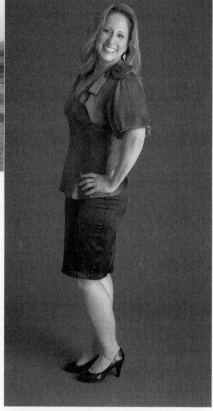

I took a long, hard look at my diet and lost 110 pounds.

by Melissa Benavides

Growing up in San Antonio, I savored the Mexican dishes that my family ate— enchiladas smothered in cheese, tacos stuffed with meat—not to mention lots of cookies and cake. But it wasn't until I got married and had two children that my weight spiraled out of control. I gained 60 pounds with each pregnancy, and although I tried several diets, I always gained it all back.

Between work and kids, I didn't have time to cook, so I picked up burgers, pizza, and, of course, Mexican for lunch and dinner. Whenever I felt sluggish, I opened a soda. At one point, I was drinking a six-pack a day! By age 37, I weighed 250 pounds. I had asthma, my knees ached, and I suffered constant headaches. Even worse, I couldn't play with my children. When I offered to walk my older son to school, he'd decline. It broke my heart that he was ashamed to be seen with me.

Small Steps, Big Impact

When my father was diagnosed with colon cancer, it finally hit me: If I continued on this path, I might not see my kids grow up. It terrified me. That's when I happened to read a magazine article about a woman who slimmed down at a local LA Weight Loss Center. The program sounded simple: Meet with a counselor weekly and learn about portion control and smart substitutions. Best of all, the plan didn't have its own brand of required food. I loved that.

I worried that I'd hate my new lifestyle, but I discovered I didn't mind trading soda for water or cutting back on sweets. I began eating more salads, fish, and baked chicken, and I even learned to cook leaner and lighter versions of my beloved Mexican fare that were surprisingly satisfying.

Total Transformation

Today, I'm 110 pounds lighter, and my weight loss has brought my family closer. When my kids want to play soccer in the park, I race them there. And now my son asks me to walk him to school. My doctor says I've added 10 years to my life. Knowing that my hard work has given me extra time with my family is what thrills me the most.

Here are my top tips.

MODIFY YOUR FAVORITES. I didn't want to give up Mexican food, so I lightened it with low-fat cheese, whole wheat tortillas, and sautéed vegetables.

PRACTICE SELF-REFLECTION. Keep a food journal and analyze it every night. If you've gotten off course, you can make an adjustment the next day.

CARRY BACK-UP SNACKS. I used to grab fast food when the hunger pangs hit. Now I have healthy, portion-controlled snacks in plastic bags on hand at all times so I don't blow my diet.

DON'T ARRIVE HUNGRY. To avoid overindulging at events, I fill up on fruits and veggies before I head out. Then I have just a taste of dessert later on.

APPRECIATE FEELING ENERGIZED. When I lost the weight, all of my health problems—the headaches, sore knees, and asthma—disappeared, too. In their place: immense self-confidence!

Part 3

FITNESS MOVES

CHAPTER 12

The Workouts Your
BODY CRAVES

If your body could tell you the best routines to melt fat fast, what would it say? According to new research, these three workouts—all 20 minutes or less—have the edge when it comes to faster, more efficient weight loss.

What if we told you that you could get all the better-body benefits of a half-hour workout in just 8 minutes? Sound too good to be true? We thought so, too, until we talked to the experts. The secret is supercharged, high-intensity interval training, which is a shorter but revved-up version of typical interval workouts. In fact, scientists are so excited about these new findings that the American College of Sports Medicine hosted a special session on the topic at its latest conference. Try one—or all—of our speedy routines, ranging from 8 to 20 minutes.

In just 2 weeks, you'll see a fitter, firmer body. Keep it up to flatten your belly, slim your thighs, and even drop a size this month—without dieting.

C raig Ballantyne, a Toronto-based exercise physiologist and strength coach who specializes in interval routines, designed the workouts.

WHY INTERVALS SLIM FASTER

Introducing short bouts of vigorous activity can speed up weight loss and cut your workout time by up to half or more. Australian researchers found that women who alternated just 8 seconds of high-intensity exercise with 12 seconds of low-intensity activity for 20 minutes, 3 times a week, slimmed down faster than steady-paced exercisers who worked out twice as long. Those who did intervals lost up to 16 pounds, shrunk their bellies by 12 percent and their thighs by 15 percent, and gained, on average, $1\frac{1}{2}$ pounds of metabolism-revving muscle in 4 months—without dieting.

Intervals increase calorie burn both during and after exercise, which helps you lose weight faster. They might also work on a biochemical level. Vigorous activity normally produces lactate, which is a by-product of the breakdown of carbs for energy that inhibits fat burning, says lead author E. Gail Trapp, PhD, exercise science researcher at the University of New South Wales, Australia. It appears that by doing supershort bouts, lactate production is reduced to blast fat more effectively. At the same time, interval workouts may increase adrenaline, a hormone that helps burn belly fat.

WORKOUTS AT A GLANCE

What you'll need: Supportive athletic shoes (specifically running ones if that's what you're doing), a watch with a second hand or timer, a cardio machine for Workout 2.

What to do: Choose one of our supercharged high-intensity interval workouts—or mix and match them—and perform it 3 times a week on nonconsecutive days.

How to do it: During low-intensity portions, you should be able to carry on a conversation easily. When you kick it into high gear, push yourself to the point that talking is nearly impossible.

"Research shows that just about anyone—including people with heart disease, diabetes, or obesity—can safely benefit from vigorous, short bouts," says Martin Gibala, PhD, professor and chair of the Department of Kinesiology at McMaster University in Ontario.

If you have any health conditions or don't exercise regularly, check with your doctor before trying these routines.

For faster results: Add traditional cardio and strength workouts to your schedule. See "Drop Pounds Even Faster!" on page 160.

Workout 1: 8-Minute Energy Booster

When McMaster University researchers had adults do four 30-second sprints (that's just 2 minutes of intense exercise!) on stationary bikes with easy pedaling in between, 3 days a week, they doubled their fitness capacity (the strength of their heart, lungs, and arteries) after 6 weeks and reported feeling stronger, firmer, and more energetic in just 2 weeks.

Our 8-minute workout, based on this study, delivers the same powerful 2 minutes of vigorous activity but in shorter bouts—15 seconds each—so you can really give it your all for faster results. For variety and to work different muscles, try this routine using the Fat-Blaster Moves (page 161) from Workout 3.

MINUTES	ACTIVITY
0:00	Warm up, walking at a moderate pace
2:00	Sprint, running as fast as you can
2:15	Walk at an easy pace
2:45	Sprint
3:00	Walk
3:30	Alternate 15-second sprint and 30-second walk intervals 6 more times
8:00	Finish

Workout 2: 12-Minute Calorie Burner

Here's an indoor alternative to the 8-minute routine that delivers the same fabulous results. You can use any cardio machine, including a treadmill, an elliptical, or a stationary bike. The session and intervals are slightly longer (12 minutes total with 20- and 40-second intervals) to allow time for the equipment to adjust to the different intensity levels.

MINUTES	ACTIVITY
0:00	Warm up by going at an easy pace
2:00	Rev it up, increasing speed, incline, or resistance so you're pushing yourself really hard
2:20	Take it easy, decreasing speed, incline, or resistance so you're going at a comfortable, moderate pace
3:00	Rev it up
3:20	Take it easy
4:00	Alternate 20-second rev-it-up and 40-second take-it-easy intervals 7 more times
11:00	Cool down by going at an easy pace
12:00	Finish

DROP POUNDS EVEN FASTER!

DO MORE CARDIO. Aim for 30 to 45 minutes of moderate, steady-paced, aerobic activity, such as walking, 2 or 3 times a week on non-interval days. You'll boost calorie burn and give your body time to recover from the higher-intensity workouts.

HIT THE WEIGHTS. Do 2 or 3 strength-training workouts on nonconsecutive days. You'll see a firmer body and a revved-up metabolism (see www.prevention.com/strengthroutine).

Workout 3: 20-Minute Fat Blaster

This high-energy plan will reshape your body in no time. The simple Fat-Blasting Moves beginning on page 162 make it doable almost anywhere. We've matched the interval ratio from the study, but the bouts are slightly longer (12 and 18 seconds) to allow you to transition between moves and still hit your peak effort level to burn maximum fat. Marching in place is an easy way to recover in between. For a challenge, try this routine alternating sprints and walking like in Workout 1.

MINUTES	ACTIVITY
0:00	Warm up by walking around or marching in place
2:00	Jumping Jacks (p. 162)
2:12	March in place
2:30	Speed Skater (p. 162)
2:42	March in place
3:00	High Knees (p. 163)
3:12	March in place
3:30	Twist (p. 163)
3:42	March in place
4:00	Repeat above intervals 7 more times in the order listed
18:00	Cool down by walking around or marching in place
20:00	Finish

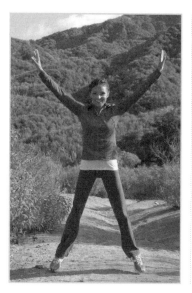

⊙ JUMPING JACKS

Yep, the ones you used to do in PE class. Go as fast as you can.

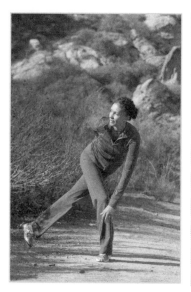

⊙ SPEED SKATER

Stand with feet together, arms at sides. Jump to right, leading with right leg. Left leg follows and crosses behind right foot as you land. Simultaneously reach left arm across body as if trying to touch floor. Repeat to left. Jump side to side as quickly as possible.

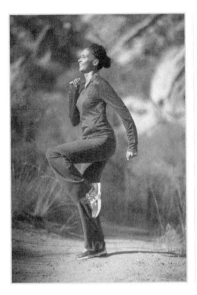

$\langle$ HIGH KNEES

Run in place as fast as you can, lifting knees out in front of you as high as possible. Swing arms at sides.

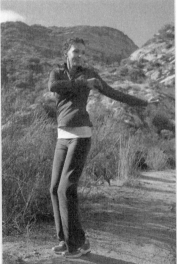

$\langle$ TWIST

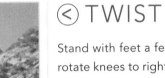

Stand with feet a few inches apart. Hop and rotate knees to right as arms go to left, landing with knees bent. Repeat, twisting in opposite direction.

CHAPTER 13

The Trouble-Zone
SHRINKER

Strength training is the quickest way to firm. Our breakthrough routine powers up metabolism and triples results.

Say farewell to flab! You *can* still firm your arms, abs, butt, and thighs. Our plan, based on new research from Ithaca College, triples your toning results and scorches over 500 calories per session. Grab an exercise band and a set of dumbbells, a combo that scientists found provided 3 times the sculpting power of ordinary weight routines. According to study author Gary Sforzo, PhD, your muscles typically work their hardest during only one part of each move, but adding bands keeps the pressure on from start to finish for significantly faster sculpting.

Our total body workout pairs this unique technique with moves to tackle all your trouble spots. Plus, we've added cardio bursts to keep your calorie burn high, and fun activities that let you melt fat while enjoying time with friends and family. The end result: You'll lose inches all over, give your metabolism a major boost, sculpt sexy muscles, and drop up to two sizes in 2 weeks—without dieting!

WORKOUT AT A GLANCE

What you'll need: A mat, a pair of 3- to 5-pound dumbbells, and a 5-foot resistance band ($5, www.spri.com; go to "Shop By: As Seen in Prevention").

3 times a week: Do the 50-minute Triple Toning Circuit (see opposite page) on nonconsecutive days. This pairs total body-sculpting moves using the band-dumbbell combo with heart-pumping cardio bursts to send your metabolism soaring. (For tips on how to use the band and dumbbell correctly, see below.)

3 or 4 times a week: Pick a Calorie Blaster (see page 172) to keep your body in fat-burning mode 24-7 and prevent boredom.

HOW TO USE RESISTANCE BANDS

A stretchy band is the simplest, most effective toning tool you can fit in your pocket. Here's a quick guide to help you get a better workout.

CHOOSE THE RIGHT WEIGHT. Start with a medium-weight band. To increase the resistance, fold it lengthwise or shorten the band by holding it closer to the anchor. To make it easier, attach one end to an anchor point instead of looping it and hold the other end in your hand.

ANCHOR IT CORRECTLY. For some moves, you need a sturdy place to hold the center or one end of a band. To anchor up high, you can buy a door attachment for less than $5, or simply put a knot in the band and close it in a door. For a low anchor, slide it under a piece of furniture or loop it around a sturdy object such as a couch leg. Make sure the band is taut when you begin a move.

COMBINE WITH DUMBBELLS. The easiest way is simply to hold the band and dumbbell together in one or both hands. If you're not able to get a good grip, tie the band around the middle of the dumbbell.

USE PROPER TECHNIQUE. Control is key to maximizing toning and avoiding injury. Don't let the band snap back once you've reached the top of the move; pause, then release slowly, resisting against the band's pull.

For even faster results: Cut 250 calories a day from your diet to boost your weight loss by about 50 percent.

Triple Toning Circuit

TIME	ACTIVITY
0:00	Warmup: March in place
5:00	Move 1: Overhead Lift (page 168) (15–20 reps)
5:45	Cardio burst: Jog or jump in place
6:45	Move 2: Lunge Repeater (page 168) (10–12 reps per side)
7:30	Cardio burst
8:30	Move 3: Sword Draw (page 169) (10–12 reps per side)
9:15	Cardio burst
10:15	Move 4: Tabletop Balance (page 169) (10–12 reps per side)
11:00	Cardio burst
12:00	Move 5: Scissor Press (page 170) (10–12 reps per side)
12:45	Cardio burst
13:45	Move 6: Power Wood Chop (page 170) (10–12 reps per side)
14:30	Cardio burst
15:30	Move 7: Chest-Press Crunch (page 171) (15–20 reps)
16:15	Cardio burst
17:15	Move 8: Knee-Up Row (page 171) (10–12 reps per side)
18:00	Cardio burst
19:00	Repeat minutes 5:00–19:00 twice
47:00	Cooldown: March in place
50:00	Finish

OUR EXPERT

Fred Engelfried, a certified instructor and 2009 Trainer of the Year at the Sports Club/LA in Los Angeles, developed this routine.

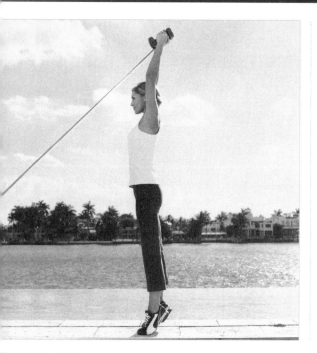

⊙ OVERHEAD LIFT

FIRMS SHOULDERS, BACK, BUTT, LEGS

Stand with feet shoulder-width apart, band anchored at ground height in front of you. Hold ends of band and a dumbbell with both hands. Bend knees and hips to sit back into a squat (keep knees behind toes), arms outstretched at waist height. Stand up as you raise hands overhead and lift heels off floor. Pause, then lower to squat again. Do 15 to 20 reps.

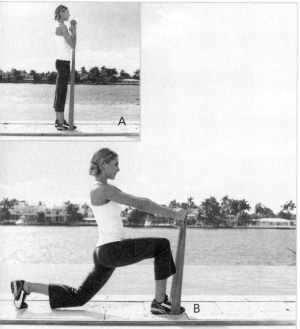

⊙ LUNGE REPEATER

FIRMS BICEPS, HIPS, BUTT, THIGHS

Stand with feet hip-width apart, center of band under right foot. Hold one end of band and a dumbbell in each hand, arms at sides, palms facing in. Bend elbows and curl hands toward shoulders, rotating arms so palms face chest (A). Straighten arms and take a big step backward with left leg, bending both knees to lower into a lunge with right knee directly over ankle, arms extended to front (B). Step back to start and repeat. Do 10 to 12 reps per side.

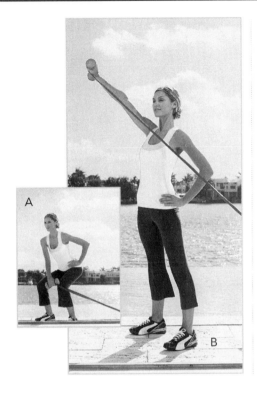

< SWORD DRAW

FIRMS SHOULDERS, BACK, ARMS, FRONT AND SIDES OF ABS, BUTT, THIGHS

Stand to right of band anchored near ground, one end of band and dumbbell in right hand at left hip. Slowly sit back into a squat, rotating torso slightly left (A). Stand, pulling band across body toward upper right, arm straight (B). Return to start. Do 10 to 12 reps per side.

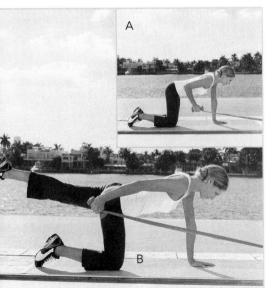

< TABLETOP BALANCE

FIRMS ARMS, ABS, BUTT

Start on hands and knees with back straight, abs pulled in. Hold a dumbbell and one end of band, anchored at ground height in front, in right hand with arm bent 90 degrees and elbow by side (A). As you straighten right arm and press dumbbell back, extend left leg straight back, squeezing glutes (B). Slowly lower leg and dumbbell. Do 10 to 12 reps per side.

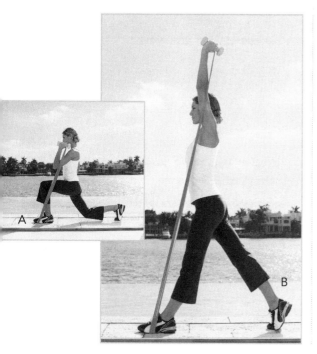

< SCISSOR PRESS

FIRMS SHOULDERS, BACK, BUTT, HIPS, THIGHS

Stand with feet in a split stance, left foot about 2 feet in front of right. Anchor one end of band under left foot and hold other end along with dumbbell in left hand at shoulder height (palm facing in). Bend both knees to about 90 degrees (A). Straighten to stand, simultaneously pressing dumbbell straight overhead (B). Lower dumbbell as you bend knees. Do 10 to 12 reps per side.

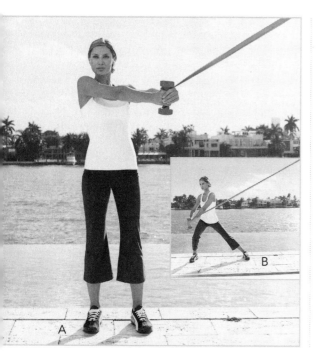

< POWER WOOD CHOP

FIRMS FRONT AND SIDES OF ABS, BUTT, INNER AND OUTER THIGHS

Anchor band overhead and stand to right side of anchor point. Hold band and dumbbell with both hands in front of you (A). Step sideways with right foot and bend only that knee into a side lunge (both feet pointing forward) while rotating torso to right and pulling band down toward right hip (B). Return to start. Do 10 to 12 reps per side.

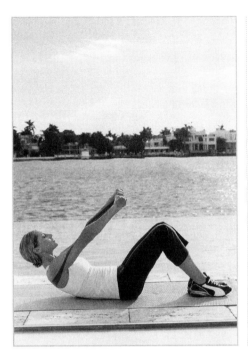

< CHEST-PRESS CRUNCH

FIRMS CHEST, ABS

Lie with knees bent, feet flat on floor, band centered under upper back. Hold one end of band and a dumbbell in each hand at chest level, elbows bent to sides. Press arms straight overhead. Keeping arms straight, contract abs to raise head and shoulders off floor. Lower to start. Do 15 to 20 reps.

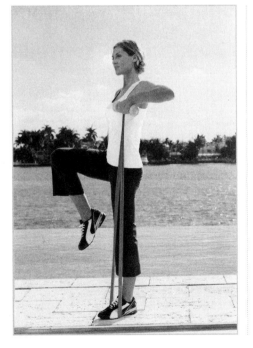

< KNEE-UP ROW

FIRMS SHOULDERS, BACK, HIPS

With band anchored under left foot, hold dumbbell and both ends of band in left hand, arm down and slightly forward. Stand on left foot, right leg extended behind you, toes just touching floor. Bend elbow to pull left hand toward chest while raising right knee to hip height or higher. Return to start. Do 10 to 12 reps per side.

13 SUPER CALORIE BLASTERS

Burn fat without missing out on fun! Try these activities 3 or 4 times a week to effortlessly amp up your weight loss and stay motivated.

ACTIVITY	CALORIES BURNED PER HOUR*
Grab a pal for a game of tennis	544
Play beach volleyball with the family	544
Swim laps while the kids splash each other	476
Go for a bike ride	476
Take a hike	442
Join the office softball game	340
Paddle off on a canoeing excursion	340
Play golf (and carry your own clubs!)	306
Catch up on your gardening	306
Go horseback riding	272
Stroll around town	238
Throw a Frisbee	204
Learn to sail	204

* Calorie burn based on a 150-pound person

THE BEST CARDIO MOVES

Here are some of our favorite ways to tone up on top and burn fat all over.

SWIMMING. The water doesn't just cool you off: It provides full-body resistance you don't encounter on land. Your arms are key for propelling you forward, so you'll sculpt strong, sleek swimmer's arms while burning as many as 680 calories an hour.

CARDIO MACHINES WITH MOVABLE HANDLES. Focus on pushing and pulling with every stride. Start by doing 1 minute with arms/1 minute without, and gradually increase. If your machine doesn't have handles, bend your elbows and pump your arms as though you're power walking.

ROCK CLIMBING. Grasping overhead handholds gives your upper body a fresh workout, and you can blast up to 750 calories an hour as you figure out the best route to the top. Find indoor climbing facilities nationwide at www.indoorclimbing.com.

KICKBOXING CLASSES. Throwing punches and jabs is a great way to get your heart pumping and melt up to 680 calories an hour. Get two free 20-minute routines to try at www.exercisetv.tv (click on "Kick Boxing").

CANOEING OR KAYAKING. Paddling down a river is the perfect family adventure, and it burns up to about 500 calories an hour.

WALKING WITH POLES. Studies show it can boost your calorie burn by more than 20 percent without making your walk feel any harder. Find poles and more info at www.walkingpoles.com.

CHAPTER 14

The Essential Over-40
WORKOUT

If there's a secret weapon for fighting midlife weight, this is it. Follow it and rev your metabolism, firm up all over, and stay lean for life.

If you're over 40, losing weight is not as hard as you think. Although strength training is key, new research shows that how you train can make a difference between so-so results and a metabolism that stays in high gear, burning fat and showing off lean muscle. The secret is targeting a specific type of muscle fiber called type II, or fast-twitch, that's responsible for bursts of speed and power. This type of muscle, as the name implies, is faster as well as denser, a combo that may yield quicker results.

These essential fibers, however, are the first to go as you get older (even if you're active), because most workouts don't target them. If you don't use them, you lose them.

Fortunately, there's an easy antidote: speed. Research from Salisbury University in Maryland found that lifting weights faster recruits more muscle and increases calorie burn by about 32 percent. That's 72 extra calories per workout, which is the amount you'd burn walking a mile! The best part: You may feel stronger after just one workout. Combine it with our plan below to firm up your toughest trouble zones and drop a size this month.

WORKOUT AT A GLANCE

What you'll need: One 6-foot flat exercise band (or two shorter ones tied together), medium resistance (available at sporting goods stores or www.spri.com).

3 days a week: Do the 30-minute Speed Training Strength Plan on below. Perform 3 sets of 8 reps of each exercise in the order listed, resting 30 seconds between sets, then repeat the entire routine one more time. Also do the 30-minute Speed Training Cardio Moves on page 182 to fire up any dozing fast-twitch fibers in those hard-to-hit lower-body areas like your hips, butt, and thighs.

The rest of the week: Do 30 to 60 minutes of any type of moderate-intensity cardio—such as walking—as many days as possible to keep your metabolism revved and speed your weight loss.

For faster results: Limit your calorie intake to 1,600 calories a day. For most women, that's a reduction of about 400 calories, which could double your weight loss. For calorie-cutting tips, see page 181.

SPEED TRAINING STRENGTH PLAN

Exercise bands are ideal for fast lifting because they provide just the right amount of resistance for great results without risking injury from hoisting heavy weights at high speed. Here's how to speed train: Perform the lifting part of each move as quickly as possible, using forceful, fast contractions of 1 count while maintaining control and good form. Return to start position at a slower 3-count pace. Adjust your hand position on the band to ensure it's taut throughout each move for the most resistance and faster toning.

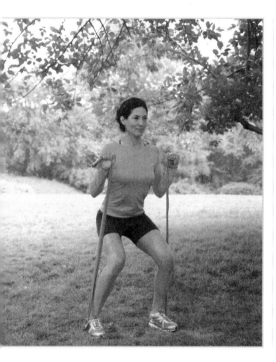

⊙ SLINGSHOT SQUAT

FIRMS BUTT AND LEGS

Stand on band with feet shoulder-width apart. Hold ends at shoulder height, palms forward. Bend hips and knees and sit back, keeping knees behind toes. This is the start position. Quickly (1 count) stand up, then slowly (3 counts) lower.

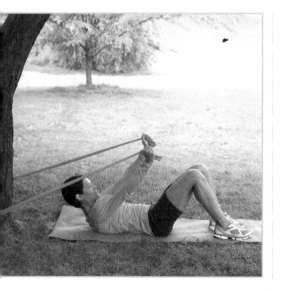

⊙ CRUNCH & PRESS

FIRMS TRICEPS AND ABS

Loop band around a sturdy object near the ground. Lie with band behind you, knees bent, feet flat. Hold each end of band and bend arms so elbows point up with hands above shoulders. Quickly curl head and shoulders off ground, then rapidly extend arms so they are straight out from shoulders. Slowly return to start position.

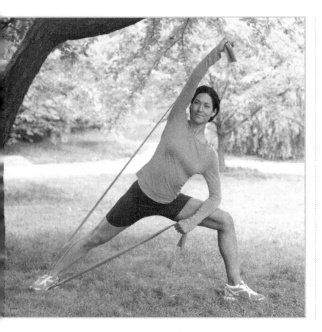

⊙ TRIANGLE PRESS

FIRMS SHOULDERS

Place right foot on center of band, holding ends in each hand. Step left foot about 3 feet to left, turn foot out, and bend knee into side lunge, keeping right leg straight. Rest left forearm on left thigh, and bend right arm so hand is by right shoulder. Quickly press right arm overhead on a diagonal. Slowly lower. Complete a full set, then switch sides.

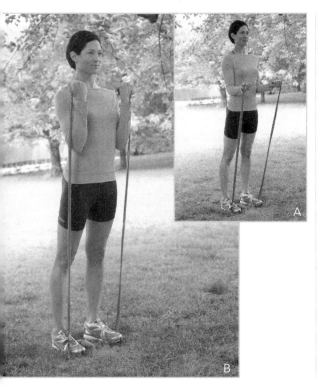

⊙ HALF CURL

FIRMS BICEPS

Stand on band with feet a few inches apart. Hold ends with arms bent 90 degrees, elbows at sides, palms up (A). Quickly bend elbows, raising hands toward shoulders (B). Slowly lower to start.

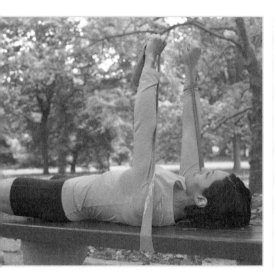

⊙ BENCH PRESS

FIRMS CHEST

Loop band underneath a bench or aerobic step and grasp one end of band in each hand. Lie back with knees bent, feet flat, and hands by chest, elbows pointing slightly down and out. Quickly straighten arms toward sky without locking elbows. Slowly lower.

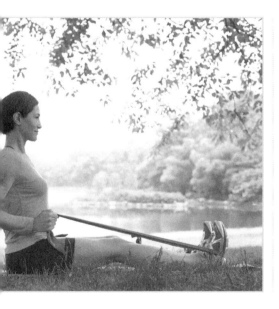

⊙ SEATED ROW

FIRMS BACK

Sit with knees bent slightly and feet flexed, heels resting on ground. Loop band around feet and grasp an end in each hand. Keeping back straight, quickly bend arms and pull hands toward rib cage, elbows pointing behind you. Slowly extend arms.

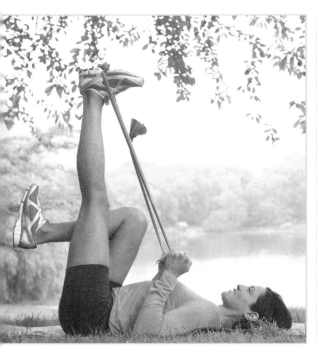

ⓒ LEG PRESS

FIRMS BUTT AND THIGHS

Lie on back with legs bent in toward chest. Loop band around bottom of left foot, with sole facing up, and grasp ends of band. Quickly straighten left leg, without locking knee. Slowly return to start position. Complete a full set, then switch legs.

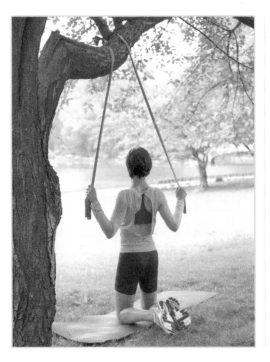

ⓒ LAT PULL-DOWN

FIRMS BACK

Loop band overhead. (To attach in a door, put a knot in center of band, drape knot over door so loose ends are on your side, close door, and check that band is secure.) Kneel facing band, arms extended overhead, hands wider than shoulder-width apart. Quickly pull hands down, squeezing shoulder blades together, until hands are around chest height. Slowly release.

FIVE CALORIE CUTTERS TO FIGHT OVER-40 FAT

Recent research confirms that the most important component for weight loss, especially after age 40, is controlling calories. Aim for 1,600 daily for optimal weight loss. To help, we rounded up the best research-backed tips for cutting calories, curbing your appetite, and keeping your weight loss efforts on the fast track.

WATCH HOME-COOKED PORTIONS. Restaurant servings aren't the only ones growing. According to a study of 18 recipes published in *The Joy of Cooking* since it was first released in 1936, home-cooked meals have 63 percent more calories per serving today. One of the reasons is a 33 percent increase in serving sizes since 1996. The solution: halve the recipes. Or assume you'll have leftovers and store half the food as soon as it's cooked.

SKIP THE SWEET DRINKS. People who eliminated just one sugar-sweetened beverage from their diets a day lost more weight over 6 months than those who reduced the same number of calories from solid food, found a Johns Hopkins University study. Researchers speculate that liquid calories are less satiating, leaving you hungrier.

EAT PROTEIN AT EVERY MEAL (AND SNACK). In a European study of 205 slimmed-down men and women, those who ate about 25 percent of their daily calories from protein (about 100 grams for a 1,600-calorie diet) had an easier time maintaining their weight loss. Protein may help because it keeps you feeling full longer and uses more calories during digestion than carbohydrates and fat do, concluded the researchers. Good choices: 3 ounces of chicken (26 grams of protein), 3 ounces of tuna (22 grams), ½ cup of low-fat cottage cheese (14 grams), ½ cup of soybeans (11 grams), 1 cup of quinoa (8 grams).

BEGIN WITH BROTH. Research shows you'll eat about 20 percent fewer calories if you start a meal with soup instead of diving right in to the main course. Just skip high-calorie creamy-based varieties.

HAVE A V8. Vegetable juice may help quell your appetite and control calorie consumption. When researchers had a group of men and women follow a low-calorie, heart-healthy diet, those who drank at least 8 ounces of low-sodium vegetable juice daily lost 4 times more weight than those who skipped the healthy beverage.

Certified personal trainer Selene Yeager, coauthor of *Move a Little, Lose a Lot,* designed the band workout. Certified fitness instructor Leigh Crews, a spokesperson for the American Council on Exercise, created the cardio routine.

SPEED TRAINING CARDIO MOVES

This 30-minute workout shapes up fast-twitch fibers—and your legs and butt—with speed or climbing intervals. To meet the intense demands, your body has to recruit all those power and speed-producing fast-twitch fibers to keep you moving.

For instance, walking uphill activates 25 percent more fibers in your backside than strolling on flat terrain, for faster sculpting. Plus it revs up calorie burn by over one-third. You can do this routine on any cardio equipment (increase the resistance on a stationary bike to simulate hills), or walk, jog, cycle, or swim outdoors. The key is to really push yourself on the speed-up/ climb intervals.

TIME	WHAT TO DO	HOW HARD*
0 to 5 min	Warm up to moderately tough pace	5 to 7
5 to 5:30	Speed up, going as fast as you can, or climb, raising incline as high as comfortably possible (10–15%)	9
5:30 to 6:30	Recover	5 to 6
6:30 to 7	Speed up or climb	9
7 to 8	Recover	5 to 6
8 to 8:30	Speed up or climb	9
8:30 to 12	Recover, then work back to moderately tough pace	5 to 7
12 to 12:45	Speed up or climb	9
12:45 to 13:45	Recover	5 to 6
13:45 to 14:30	Speed up or climb	9
14:30 to 15:30	Recover	5 to 6
15:30 to 16:15	Speed up or climb	9
16:15 to 20	Recover, then work back to moderately tough pace	5 to 7
20 to 21	Speed up or climb	9
21 to 22	Recover	5 to 6
22 to 23	Speed up or climb	9
23 to 24	Recover	5 to 6
24 to 25	Speed up or climb	9
25 to 30	Cool down	5 to 6

*Based on a scale of 1 to 10, with 1 being the effort required for sitting and 10 for an all-out sprint

CHAPTER 15

The Yes-You-Can-Run Plan

Turn your walk into a run and drop a size in 4 weeks.

We know you love walking, and we do, too! It's one of the best ways to stay healthy and keep your waistline in check. But when you're short on time (and who isn't?) or stuck on a plateau, running is another do-anywhere, no-equipment-required alternative that ramps up weight loss.

WORKOUT AT A GLANCE

What you need: Running shoes. While it's fine to walk in running shoes, it's not safe to run in walking shoes because they're designed to absorb less impact.

3 days a week: Do run/walk intervals (see chart on page 187) and Run Strong stretches (B moves only, page 191).

3 alternate days: Do 30 to 60 minutes of any low-impact cardio (such as walking, biking, or swimming) plus the Run Strong toning moves and stretches (A and B moves, page 191).

anny Dreyer, the coauthor of *Chi Running* who specializes in teaching beginners how to run pain-free, created the walk/run plan. Vonda Wright, MD, an orthopedic surgeon and author of *Fitness After 40,* designed the strength/stretching workout.

. . . .

Customize your workout: Don't want to run full-time? Stop at whatever week feels good to you. To step it up after week 8, add 5 minutes a week until you reach 60 minutes.

Adding even a few minutes onto your walks can build stronger bones and cut your exercise time nearly in half: Minute for minute, running burns about twice as many calories as walking.

But if you think you're too old or too out of shape or that running will damage your knees (research shows it won't), don't take it from us. Take it from the 46-to-67-year-old women who tested our walk-to-run program: They saw pounds disappear as soon as the first week, and by 8 weeks, they had shaved up to 20 inches off their butts, thighs, waistlines, hips, and arms and dropped nearly 3 sizes—all without dieting! In fact, even those who didn't lose much weight erased as many as 5 inches of belly fat.

Our 8-week plan is specifically designed to be safe for would-be runners over 40. You'll gradually increase your running time, allowing your body to adjust without aches or strain, and perform targeted toning exercises and stretches to protect against injuries. And don't be surprised if you become a convert. Adults in one study who tried jogging reported enjoying their workouts 30 percent more than when they walked, possibly because running stimulates more good-mood hormones in the brain, say researchers.

YOUR 8-WEEK TRAINING PLAN

Before and after every workout, do 4 minutes of easy walking to warm up and cool down. You can rearrange days as needed, but don't run on back-to-back days. Ditto for toning moves.

Week 1

DAY	WORKOUT
Monday	Run 1 min/walk 3 min; do 13 times (total 60 min)
Tuesday	Low-impact cardio; Run Strong moves (A & B)
Wednesday	Repeat Monday's routine
Thursday	Low-impact cardio; Run Strong moves (A & B)
Friday	Repeat Monday's routine
Saturday	Low-impact cardio; Run Strong moves (A & B)
Sunday	Rest

Week 2

DAY	WORKOUT
Monday	Run 3 min/walk 2 min; do 8 times (total 48 min)
Tuesday	Low-impact cardio; Run Strong moves (A & B)
Wednesday	Run 3 min/walk 1 min; do 8 times (total 40 min)
Thursday	Low-impact cardio; Run Strong moves (A & B)
Friday	Repeat Wednesday's routine
Saturday	Low-impact cardio; Run Strong moves (A & B)
Sunday	Rest

Week 3

DAY	WORKOUT
Monday	Run 5 min/walk 3 min; do 6 times (total 56 min)
Tuesday	Low-impact cardio; Run Strong moves (A & B)
Wednesday	Run 5 min/walk 2 min; do 6 times (total 50 min)
Thursday	Low-impact cardio; Run Strong moves (A & B)
Friday	Run 5 min/walk 1 min; do 6 times (total 44 min)
Saturday	Low-impact cardio; Run Strong moves (A & B)
Sunday	Rest

Week 4

DAY	WORKOUT
Monday	Run 8 min/walk 3 min; do 3 times (total 41 min)
Tuesday	Low-impact cardio; Run Strong moves (A & B)
Wednesday	Run 8 min/walk 2 min; do 3 times (total 38 min)
Thursday	Low-impact cardio; Run Strong moves (A & B)
Friday	Run 8 min/walk 1 min; do 3 times (total 35 min)
Saturday	Low-impact cardio; Run Strong moves (A & B)
Sunday	Rest

Week 5

DAY	WORKOUT
Monday	Run 10 min/walk 3 min; do 3 times (total 47 min)
Tuesday	Low-impact cardio; Run Strong moves (A & B)
Wednesday	Run 10 min/walk 2 min; do 3 times (total 44 min)
Thursday	Low-impact cardio; Run Strong moves (A & B)
Friday	Run 10 min/walk 1 min; do 3 times (total 41 min)
Saturday	Low-impact cardio; Run Strong moves (A & B)
Sunday	Rest

Week 6

DAY	WORKOUT
Monday	Run 15 min/walk 2 min; do 2 times (total 42 min)
Tuesday	Low-impact cardio; Run Strong moves (A & B)
Wednesday	Repeat Monday's routine
Thursday	Low-impact cardio; Run Strong moves (A & B)
Friday	Run 15 min/walk 1 min; do 2 times (total 40 min)
Saturday	Low-impact cardio; Run Strong moves (A & B)
Sunday	Rest

Week 7

DAY	WORKOUT
Monday	Run 20 min/walk 2 min/run 10 min (total 40 min)
Tuesday	Low-impact cardio; Run Strong moves (A & B)
Wednesday	Repeat Monday's routine
Thursday	Low-impact cardio; Run Strong moves (A & B)
Friday	Run 20 min/walk 1 min/run 10 min (total 39 min)
Saturday	Low-impact cardio; Run Strong moves (A & B)
Sunday	Rest

Week 8

DAY	WORKOUT
Monday	Run 25 min/walk 2 min/run 5 min (total 40 min)
Tuesday	Low-impact cardio; Run Strong moves (A & B)
Wednesday	Run 25 min/walk 1 min/run 5 min (total 39 min) Low-impact cardio; Run Strong moves (A & B)
Thursday	Low-impact cardio; Run Strong moves (A & B)
Friday	Run 30 min! Low-impact cardio; Run Strong moves (A & B)
Saturday	Low-impact cardio; Run Strong moves (A & B)
Sunday	Rest

INJURY-PROOF YOUR RUN

Good form and technique reduce strain and help your body absorb shock for a pain-free workout. Focus on one tip below each time you run.

PROTECT YOUR POSTURE. Keep your shoulders back and down, chest lifted, abs tight. Lean your entire body slightly forward from your ankles (don't bend at the waist), allowing gravity to gently pull you forward.

KEEP YOUR EYES ON THE HORIZON. Look out ahead, rather than at the ground. Keeping your gaze up makes walking and running easier.

RELAX YOUR HANDS. Clenching your fists can send tension up your wrists and arms; loosen up by pretending to cup something fragile, such as a potato chip or butterfly.

MAKE SMOOTH TRANSITIONS. In the final seconds of each walking interval, pick up your pace so when you switch to running, it feels easier than if you tried to walk any faster.

LAND MIDFOOT. Unlike walking, striking the ground with your heel when you run puts on the brakes. Aim to come down with the middle of your foot landing under you, then roll through smoothly.

SHORTEN YOUR STRIDE. Protect your knees and absorb shock better by maintaining a short stride and keeping a slight bend in your knee as you land.

PICK YOUR FEET UP. Instead of pushing into the ground, which can fatigue muscles, focus on keeping your legs relaxed and lifting feet up.

RUN STRONG AND SLIM DOWN FASTER

Strengthening and stretching your hips, butt, and abs can help you speed up, burn more fat, and stave off injuries. Do 2 sets of 10 to 15 reps of each toning move (A) per side, 3 times a week. Hold stretches (B) for 30 seconds per side. Do stretches after run/walk workouts.

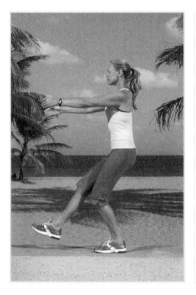

< 1A ONE-LEGGED SQUAT

TONES THIGHS AND IMPROVES KNEE FUNCTION

Balance on left leg, right foot lifted a few inches off of ground in front, arms outstretched. Keeping back straight, slowly bend right knee and sit back 2 to 3 inches. Press into left heel to stand.

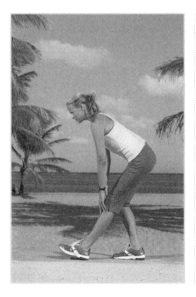

< 1B HAMSTRING STRETCH

Plant left heel on ground in front of you, leg straight, toes up. With weight on right leg, hinge forward from hips, and sit back to stretch back of left leg.

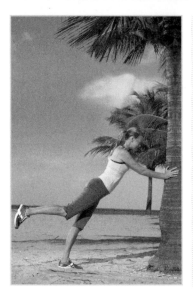

⊲ 2A LIFT AND PRESS

TONES HIPS AND BUTT FOR STRENGTH AND SPEED

Stand 3 to 4 feet away from a tree or wall. Keeping legs straight, lean forward and place palms on tree at chest height. (If you don't feel your calves stretch, walk feet back a few inches and press heels down.) Pull right knee toward chest, then press leg behind you, pushing back and up through right heel and squeezing glutes.

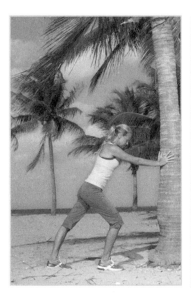

⊲ 2B CALF STRETCH

Place right foot closer to tree, right knee bent, left leg back and straight. Press hips forward until you feel a stretch in back of lower left leg.

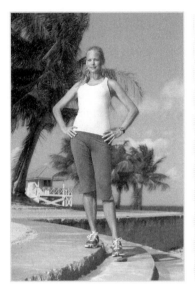

◁ 3A HIP DIP

TONES ABS AND BUTT AND IMPROVES PELVIS ALIGNMENT

Stand with right foot on a step, left one off, hips level. Stick right hip out to side, lowering left hip, leg, and foot a few inches; squeeze abs and butt to draw back up to level.

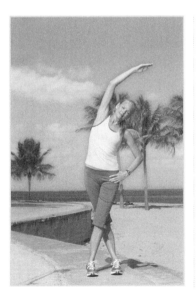

◁ 3B SIDE STRETCH

Standing on level ground, cross left leg in front of right, both feet flat, hands on hips. Reach right arm overhead, and bend body to left, pushing hips slightly to right to feel a stretch along right side of your body.

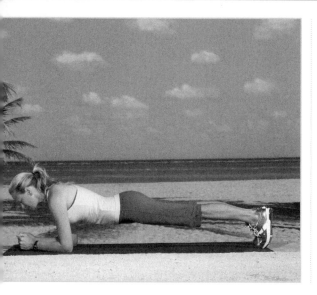

⊘ 4A PLANK

TONES CORE MUSCLES TO ENSURE GOOD POSTURE

Lie facedown on a mat, upper body propped on forearms with elbows directly beneath shoulders and toes tucked. Lift hips so body forms a straight line and you're balancing on forearms and toes. Hold for 30 seconds. Do twice.

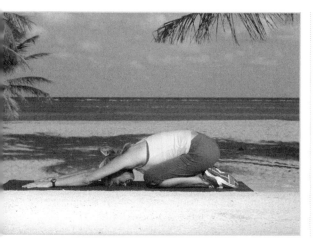

⊘ 4B BACK STRETCH

From plank position, lower knees to ground, untuck toes, and sit back on heels with arms reaching forward to stretch your torso, arms, and back.

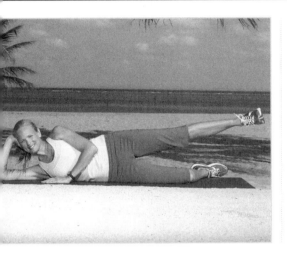

< 5A SIDE LEG LIFT

TONES OUTER THIGHS AND BUTT TO PROTECT KNEES

Lie on right side, top leg extended with foot flexed, bottom one bent behind you for balance. Bend right elbow and support head with hand. Squeeze left glute and outer thigh to raise left leg 1 to 2 feet. Pause; slowly lower to start.

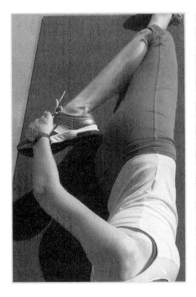

< 5B THIGH STRETCH

Lying on right side with legs stacked, bend left leg and grasp shin or forefoot with hand. Keeping left knee over right one, gently pull foot toward butt until you feel a stretch in the front of left thigh.

CHAPTER 16

Surprising Workout BLUNDERS

Avoid these six workout mistakes that slow down results.

You huff and puff through cardio sessions, but that extra layer of flab just won't budge. Surprise: Your workout might be to blame. We talked to trainers and exercise physiologists across the country and discovered six surprising ways that well-intentioned fitness routines can put the brakes on weight-loss goals.

"Many women assume that 30 minutes of exercise will change their bodies, but it's not automatic," says Geralyn Coopersmith, the director of Equinox Fitness Training Institute in New York City. "If you're focused and smart about how you use that half hour, you will be amazed by your results."

Here is what to do—and *not* to do—to rev your metabolism and slim down for good.

DON'T: SACRIFICE GOOD FORM FOR SPEED

Do: Slow down and stand tall

The results: Burn 50 extra calories per session

High-intensity exercise may burn loads of calories, but not if you're hanging on to the handrails for dear life. It's important to focus on your form, even if that means lowering the intensity.

"You recruit fewer muscles and burn fewer calories when you're slouched over," says Coopersmith. Same goes for strength training, says James Levine, MD, PhD, a scientist at the Mayo Clinic in Rochester, Minnesota, whose research has found that standing while lifting weights boosts calorie burn by about 50 calories per half hour. Best of all, one study showed that good posture allows you to take in more oxygen so your workout feels easier, even while you're blasting more calories.

DON'T: EXERCISE WHILE PARCHED

Do: Sip 15 ounces of water 2 hours before working out

The results: More energy to lift weights and firm up faster

Experts are constantly back and forth on the merits of the 8-glasses-a-day guideline. However, when it comes to working out, the importance of drinking up is clear.

"Nearly every cell in the body is composed of water. Without it, they don't function efficiently during exercise," says Dan Judelson, PhD, an assistant professor of kinesiology at California State University, Fullerton. Translation: You'll fatigue faster and your workout will feel tougher than it should.

In recent studies, Dr. Judelson discovered that exercisers who were dehydrated completed 3 to 5 fewer reps per set while strength training. Part of the problem is that dehydration decreases the body's levels of anabolic hormone that are necessary for strong muscles.

On workout days, drink an ounce of water for every 10 pounds of body weight (i.e., 15 ounces if you weigh 150) 1 to 2 hours prior to exercise. Then keep sipping during and after your session to replenish what you lose through sweat.

DON'T: READ A NOVEL ON THE TREADMILL

Do: Listen to music

The results: Burn 15 percent more calories

"If flipping through a magazine keeps you motivated, by all means do it," says Coopersmith. "But reading while exercising is so distracting that you're probably working at an intensity too low to burn a significant number of calories."

Magazines and books are just the tip of the iceberg—1 in 10 of us reads texts or e-mail on a cell phone during workouts, reports a new survey by Standard Life, a health insurance company. Instead, turn on some tunes to increase the duration and intensity of your cardio bout. Researchers at Brunel University in London discovered that runners who listened to motivational rock or pop music (think Queen or Madonna) exercised up to 15 percent longer and felt better doing it. You don't have to nix TV shows, cell phones, books, or magazines every workout. Just leave them behind a couple times a week so you can focus on intensity.

DON'T: RUN IF YOU HATE IT

Do: Pick a cardio routine that's fun

The results: Lose 4 pounds a year

No matter how many calories an activity promises to burn, if you don't enjoy it, you'll be less likely to do it and won't reap the benefits. Think of it this way: If you burn 300 calories every time you exercise, but you dread it so much that you skip one session a week, it adds up to 1,200 calories a month—or more than 4 pounds a year you won't lose. Instead, find a workout you want to do, rather than one you feel like you have to do.

When University of Nebraska at Omaha researchers polled women who'd been exercising regularly for longer than a year, they found that one of the top predictors of adherence was choosing enjoyable activities. Study author Jennifer Huberty, PhD, also suggests experimenting with ways to make exercise more appealing. For example, if walking is your workout of choice, try recruiting a friend to join you.

DON'T: PUT ALL YOUR TIME INTO CARDIO

Do: Swap aerobic exercise for weights 3 times a week

The results: Lose up to 12½ pounds in a year

More than 80 percent of women forgo strength training, says the latest survey by the Sporting Goods Manufacturers Association. If you're one of them, it may be the number one reason your scale is stuck.

You've probably heard that strength training can boost metabolism, but here's something you may not know: People who pair aerobic and resistance training eat less—517 fewer calories a day—than those who do only cardio, reports a new study in the *Journal of Sports Science and Medicine*. The combo workouts might increase satiety hormones more and boost the body's ability to break down food and stabilize blood sugar, so you feel full longer, says study author Brandon S. Shaw, PhD.

DON'T: TRUST GYM MACHINE CALORIE-BURN ESTIMATES

Do: Track your burn with a heart rate monitor

The results: Lose 3 pounds this year

Oh, how sweet it would be if 20 minutes on a cardio machine really did blast 400 calories. But like most things in life that sound too good to be true, those digital displays broadcasting mega calorie burn are often bogus.

Recent research presented at the National Strength and Conditioning Association National Conference found that elliptical trainers overestimate calorie burn by an average of 30 percent. If you're trying to create a calorie deficit to lose weight, those thought-you-burned-'em calories can add up over time and thwart your success.

To ensure you're burning the number of calories you want, consider investing in a heart rate monitor. We love the FT40 by Polar because it's a cinch to set up and use ($180; polarusa.com). Input some basic info (weight, height, age, activity level, and so on) and the gadget will accurately track your heart rate to compute the number of calories you torched. Or, for a free check of your cardio machine's readout, cross-reference your calorie burn by logging your session at www.prevention.com/fitnesstracker.

"I LOST HALF MY BODY WEIGHT!"

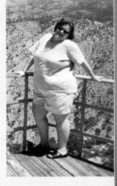

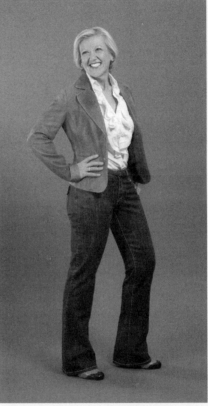

I went from an emotional eater to a three-time triathlete and lost 136 pounds.

by Sarah Montague

When I was a young girl in England, my parents went through a difficult divorce. I learned early on to medicate my feelings with food. I found comfort in feeling full and gorged myself on potato chips, chocolate, and cheese. So it's no surprise that when the pressure from my first job kicked in, I headed for the cupboard. Within 3 years, I gained 100 pounds, developed obesity-related asthma, and dislocated both knees. During that same time, I met my future husband. As we planned our wedding, it never occurred to me to try to lose the weight. Instead, I had my wedding dress custom made.

When I was 30, my husband and I moved across the Atlantic to Chicago. Within 6 months, I gained another 20 pounds. At a routine medical checkup, my doctor suggested I try Weight Watchers. I was shocked. Nobody had ever confronted me about my size, but it was the wake-up call I needed.

Good-Bye to Bingeing

I started attending weekly Weight Watchers meetings and chose 136 pounds as my goal weight. I worried that it would be too difficult to drop a lifetime of bad habits, but I counted my points carefully and paid close attention to why I was eating: emotions or hunger. I began working out, and the more weight I lost, the easier—and more fun—it became.

It took me 6 years to reach 136 pounds. Even then, I didn't consider myself athletic. So when friends approached me to train with them for a triathlon, I was hesitant. But I realized that losing so much weight was a huge accomplishment, and I needed a new challenge. I signed up for the race and finished in the middle of the pack but beaming with pride. For the first time, I was a player in the game—not a sideline spectator.

An Athlete at 40

I've competed in three triathlons so far, and when I see the athletes at these events, it still amazes me that I'm one of them. I recently turned 40, and to mark the milestone, I participated in the Chicago Triathlon, my hardest race to date. I aimed to finish in 4 hours, but I did it in 3 hours, 22 minutes. Training can be grueling, but I love working hard. I'll never numb my feelings with food again.

Here are my top tips.

THINK BEFORE YOU BITE. Before I take seconds or have dessert, I remind myself that I won't regret what I don't eat.

PLAN, PLAN, PLAN. On busy days, I always pack a lunch—otherwise, it's too likely that I'll rely on junk from the vending machines. I also stash stocked gym bags in my car and under my desk so I'm always ready to work out.

CELEBRATE SMALL VICTORIES. Competing has boosted my self-esteem, but smaller tests, such as passing on the bread basket—are just as empowering.

STICK TO A ROUTINE. I buy similar groceries weekly. That way, I get in and out with no temptation from the snack aisle.

THINK BIG PICTURE. I used to fill up without thinking about the consequences. Now I approach the week as a whole and make adjustments as needed. If I'm planning on a big dinner, I'm perfectly happy eating a light lunch.

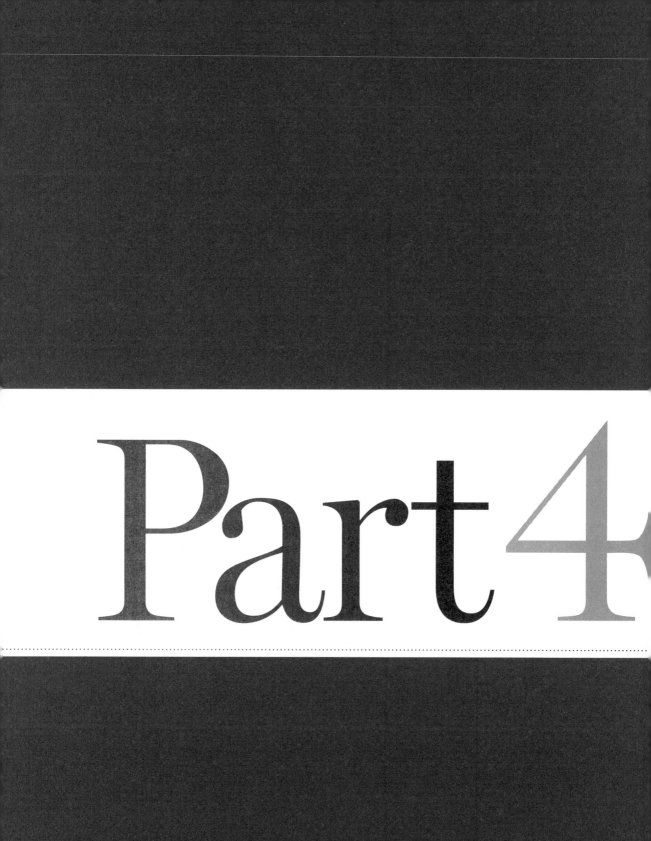

Part 4

NUTRITION
NEWS

CHAPTER 17

FOOD COMBOS
That Add Up

Make easy meals that heal with these simple additions.

Healthy eating is all about math: subtracting fat, counting calories, dividing portions. But let's not forget adding. It's the little things we toss in the pot that often yield the biggest benefits.

"Adding just one food to another can make a tremendous difference in your total nutrient intake and offer significant health gains," says Tara Gidus, RD, a spokesperson for the American Dietetic Association.

With benefits ranging from stronger bones and better eyesight to a healthier heart and improved immunity, here are 15 of our favorite quick pairings for breakfast, lunch, dinner, snacks, and even beverages that taste great, take seconds to make, and add up to amazing health.

WHOLE GRAIN CEREAL + SUNFLOWER SEEDS FOR BETTER IMMUNITY

Sprinkling $\frac{1}{2}$ cup of sunflower seeds into your morning cereal (any kind) provides more than 100 percent of your day's requirements for alpha-tocopherol, which is the most active form of vitamin E. As an antioxidant, vitamin E protects cells from damage caused by destructive free radicals that can lead to cancer and cardiovascular disease.

SCRAMBLED EGGS + RED PEPPERS FOR SMOOTHER SKIN

Tossing in $\frac{1}{2}$ cup of chopped red peppers delivers more than 100 percent of your daily vitamin C need—which spells good news for your skin. Researchers in the United Kingdom looked at vitamin C intake in 4,025 women and found that those who ate more vitamin C had less wrinkling and dryness.

SMOOTHIE + WHEAT GERM FOR FASTER HEALING OF CUTS AND BRUISES

One-quarter cup of wheat germ packs nearly half of your day's requirements for zinc, an essential mineral that helps repair cells and strengthens the immune system. Even a slight deficiency can reduce your immunity, making it harder to heal. Add it to any flavor smoothie.

SANDWICH + SPINACH LEAVES FOR DECREASED RISK OF NIGHT BLINDNESS

Stacking only three small leaves of spinach on your sandwich (any kind you'd like) satisfies at least 20 percent of your day's vitamin A requirements. Vitamin A helps you see in the dark, and it also protects your eyes from age-related macular degeneration, which can lead to vision loss.

WONDERFUL WHITES

When nutrition experts tell you to avoid "white food," they mean refined foods such as white flour, rice, and pasta. White vegetables, beans, and nuts may also lack the vibrant color connected with many disease-fighting antioxidants, but they contain surprise benefits that can lower risks of high blood pressure, heart attack, and more. Here are some great whites to try.

CAULIFLOWER: One cup of this cruciferous veggie (cooked) contains nearly 20 percent of your daily need for bone-building vitamin K. Toss florets with oil and red-pepper flakes and roast.

ONIONS: They're a rich source of quercetin, a flavonoid linked to reduced risk of colon cancer. Chop and sprinkle onto canned soups for a homemade touch.

JICAMA: A cup provides nearly one-quarter of the daily fiber requirement and one-third of your need for the antioxidant vitamin C. Slice thinly into strips and dip into salsa.

RADISHES: A peppery addition to salads, ½ cup has 9 calories and is a good source of vitamin C.

GARLIC: It may lower blood pressure and cholesterol levels and protect against cancer. Crush before using in recipes to unleash healthful compounds.

CANNELLINI BEANS: Just 1 cup provides nearly half of your daily fiber need and 14 grams of filling protein. Sauté with olive oil and rosemary for a quick side.

PARSNIPS: This carrot cousin is packed with vitamin C and fiber. Slice, drizzle with oil and maple syrup, and roast in the oven.

PINE NUTS: They're rich in manganese, a mineral crucial for metabolism and bone health. Toast and toss onto soups and salads.

GARDEN SALAD + CANNED WILD SALMON FOR HEALTHIER BRAIN AND HEART

Adding 3 ounces of canned wild salmon to your salad provides half of the weekly recommendation for healthy omega-3 fats. The fatty acids found in canned salmon are linked to improvements in heart and brain health. Choosing wild lowers your exposure to dioxin, which is a cancer-causing contaminant found in the feed given to the farm-raised variety, says Evelyn Tribole, RD, author of *The Ultimate Omega-3 Diet*.

STIR-FRY + KALE FOR STRONGER EYES

One-half cup of kale delivers at least 12 milligrams of lutein and zeaxanthin, carotenoids found in dark leafy greens that help combat cataracts and age-related macular degeneration (AMD). Results from the Eye Disease Case-Control Study found that people who ate the most of these nutrients—as much as 5.8 milligrams a day—had a significantly lower risk of AMD than those who ate the least. Stir-fry is the perfect way to throw it into the mix. If you're not a kale fan, other leafy greens such as Swiss chard and spinach offer similar benefits.

SALSA + CHICKPEAS FOR LOWER BODY WEIGHT

Adding chickpeas to a light dip such as salsa adds bulk without lots of calories and boosts your intake of protein, so you fill up faster and feel fuller. Eating chickpeas regularly may also improve your overall food choices. An Australian study published in the *Journal of the American Dietetic Association* found that people who ate ½ cup of chickpeas a day weighed a pound less and ate less food overall.

LOW-FAT PUDDING + NONFAT POWDERED MILK FOR LESS PMS

Sprinkling ⅓ cup of nonfat powdered milk into pudding satisfies 40 percent of your day's calcium and 50 to 100 percent of your vitamin D requirements, depending on your age. Research shows that the combination of calcium and vitamin D reduces the risk of developing PMS.

GREEN TEA + LEMON FOR LOWER CANCER RISK

Green tea is already rich in antioxidants, but a study from Purdue University found that adding citrus juice led to a fourfold increase in disease-fighting catechins. Lemon juice in particular preserved the most catechins, while orange, lime, and grapefruit juices were less potent but effective.

WATER + UNSWEETENED CRANBERRY JUICE FOR FEWER CAVITIES

Unsweetened cranberry juice prevents the buildup of *Streptococcus mutans,* which is the bacteria behind most cavities, by preventing them from sticking to the tooth's surface. The unsweetened juice also interferes with plaque formation. Mixing it with water helps dilute the juice's tartness.

STRAWBERRIES + NONFAT GREEK YOGURT FOR MORE MUSCLE

Greek yogurt packs twice the protein of ordinary yogurt, and protein is essential for building, repairing, and maintaining muscles, which burn more calories than fat. Strawberries add a burst of natural sweetness.

PASTA + PARSLEY FOR STRONGER BONES

Topping a pasta dish (any kind) with just six sprigs of parsley offers a fresh boost of flavor and delivers a full day's supply of vitamin K, says Marisa Moore, RD, an Atlanta-based nutritionist and American Dietetic Association spokesperson. Vitamin K is important for bone health. Studies show it helps prevent fractures and may guard against bone loss.

WAKE UP THE HEALTH POWER OF YOUR FOOD

There's nothing more nutritious than a heaping salad of colorful raw vegetables, right? Not so fast, says new research. Scientists are finding that various methods of cooking veggies—from boiling carrots to steaming broccoli—can actually boost certain nutrients.

"Some of the healthiest plant pigments in vegetables are released only when they're cooked," says Elizabeth Johnson, PhD, a scientist at the Friedman School of Nutrition Science and Policy at Tufts University. "You get more carotenoids, for example, from steamed spinach than from a spinach salad."

Raw veggies are still a great way to get vitamins and minerals, but cooking them in a specific way can release additional nutrients or preserve the health benefits while making the food tastier. Next time you assemble a hearty salad or a crudités platter, toss in some of these steamed, boiled, baked, or roasted additions.

Broccoli: Steam

RAW broccoli is high in potential cancer-fighting nutrients such as betacarotene, lutein, and flavonols.

STEAMED broccoli has higher concentrations of many carotenoids (including beta-carotene and lutein) than raw, according to a recent study in the *Journal of Agricultural and Food Chemistry*. Plus, it retains nearly 70 percent of its vitamin C and virtually all of its kaempferol, a cell-saving flavonoid.

BONUS: To maximize the nutrients you get from your broccoli, wait to wash and cut it until just before steaming, suggests Ellie Krieger, RD, author of *So Easy: Luscious Healthy Recipes for Every Meal of the Week* and host of *Healthy Appetite* on the Food Network. Washing and cutting speeds up deterioration.

Carrots: Boil Until Tender

RAW carrots are a good source of vitamin C and carotenoids, a family of antioxidants that includes beta-carotene. These contribute to good eye health and might also reduce your risk of heart attack and some forms of cancer.

BOILING makes the carotenoids 14 percent more concentrated, according to a recent study in the *Journal of Agricultural and Food Chemistry*. Dietary fiber in the cell walls of carrots traps the carotenoids, but high heat releases and concentrates the compounds, making it easier for your digestive tract to access them, explains Philipp Simon, PhD, a scientist with the USDA Vegetable Crops Research Unit. The study also found that boiling increases carrots' total antioxidant capacity (their ability to attack free radicals) while only slightly diminishing vitamin C levels.

BONUS: Add a drop of oil to your cooked carrots. The fat helps your body absorb more of the beta-carotene.

Garlic: Roast for No More Than 3 Minutes

RAW garlic contains alliinase, an enzyme with antiplatelet properties that may help reduce blood pressure and prevent blood from clotting, which decreases your risk of heart disease.

ROASTING garlic cloves (for up to 3 minutes at no more than 390°F) helps retain nearly all of their anti-platelet capabilities—with less of the odoriferous side effects of raw, say researchers at the USDA and the National University of Cuyo in Argentina. Turn off the heat after 3 minutes. By 6 minutes, garlic loses about 80 percent of its clot-busting abilities; by 10 minutes, 100 percent. And don't cook it in the microwave; that destroys the alliinase, says Dr. Simon.

BONUS: Crush or chop cloves before cooking to release even more alliinase, even as cooking times increase.

Root Vegetables: Roast with Skins On

RAW winter veggies such as potatoes, turnips, and parsnips are high in fiber and vitamins, but many are not commonly eaten raw.

ROASTING with skins intact helps retain all the nutrients. If you prefer boiling, leave the skins on (peel them after cooling, if necessary), and boil them in large chunks (preferably whole) to preserve the veggies' water-soluble nutrients, says Krieger.

(continued)

BONUS: Choose a colorful variety for added health benefits. Several studies show that root vegetables with darker skins (red potatoes) or flesh (purple sweet potatoes) have more cancer-fighting polyphenols than their lighter colored cousins.

Brussels Sprouts: Steam or Stir-Fry

RAW Brussels sprouts contain sulforaphane, which is a powerful phytochemical that helps protect against breast cancer.

STEAMING OR STIR-FRYING as quickly as possible preserves more of the cancer-fighting compounds. (Boiling Brussels sprouts causes sulforaphane to leach into the water, according to research.)

BONUS: The tough cores will cook faster and more evenly if you cut an X into the bottom of each stem.

Tomatoes: Roast with Olive Oil

RAW tomatoes are rich in lycopene, which is a carotenoid that gives this fruit its red hue. Lycopene is also a powerful antioxidant that can reduce the risk of certain cancers and heart disease.

ROASTING tomatoes causes cell walls to burst, releasing more lycopene. A recent German study published in the *British Journal of Nutrition* found that 77 percent of 198 people following a strict raw food diet had plasma lycopene levels below what's considered optimal.

BONUS: Splash cherry tomatoes with olive oil, then roast them in the oven until their skins rupture, suggests Krieger. Lycopene is fat soluble, so adding olive oil helps your body absorb it.

Asparagus: Steam Vertically

RAW, 1 cup of asparagus contains nearly 20 percent of the recommended daily intake of folate, a B vitamin that helps protect your cardiovascular and nervous systems.

Recent studies link a diet high in folate with a decreased risk of Alzheimer's disease, stroke, and heart disease. Since folate is water soluble and sensitive to heat, cooking can diminish it.

STEAMING gently in a vertical steamer keeps the fragile tips—which contain most of the water-soluble nutrients—away from the liquid. (You can also steam them in a regular pot and keep the tips out of the water.) This imparts more flavor while retaining all the benefits of raw.

BONUS: Store asparagus in a cool, dark space (the back of your produce drawer, for example) to preserve the folate, which is sensitive to heat and light.

Beets: Steam Gently

RAW beets are high in betanin, a powerful plant pigment and antioxidant that can halt free-radical damage and may even stop the growth of tumor cells in the stomach, colon, lungs, and nervous system, according to several studies.

LIGHTLY STEAMING beets retains more cancer-fighting powers, Dr. Johnson says. Betanin is highly sensitive to heat, so intense cooking methods like boiling or roasting destroy the benefits.

BONUS: Peel and chop the beets before steaming to help liberate the betanin from the tough cell walls and allow the beets to cook faster.

Onions: Bake for 5 Minutes in Foil

RAW onions are one of the best sources of quercetin, a flavonoid with anti-inflammatory powers that might help control allergies and asthma, as well as help treat Alzheimer's and Parkinson's diseases.

BAKING thick chunks wrapped in foil for 5 minutes at 390°F preserves 99.5 percent of the quercetin compounds while diminishing the bite and odor, says a 2008 USDA/National Food Research Institute study.

BONUS: Choose red or yellow onions over white; they have more flavonoids. As a general rule, the darker the color, the greater the number of antioxidants.

CHAPTER 18

Eight Condiment
CURES

Boost brainpower, protect your heart, and
prevent cancer with just a squeeze of this
and a dash of that . . .

Turns out your diet may be healthier than you think. Those little extras you love, such as ketchup on burgers or hot sauce in tacos, have hidden health benefits. New research shows that certain spices, herbs, and spreads not only boost flavor but also can help curb appetite, ease digestion, and even promote better memory. Here are eight to have on hand.

KETCHUP

Lowers risk of cardiovascular disease

Daily dose: 3 to 4 tablespoons

Lycopene—a powerful antioxidant in ketchup—may slow the process that leads to atherosclerosis, says Betty Ishida, PhD, a USDA research biologist. While all ketchup contains some lycopene, a study in the *Journal of Agricultural and Food Chemistry* found that organic versions contain up to 60 percent more per gram than conventional brands. The researchers also found that organic ketchup had the highest levels of vitamins A, C, and E.

Serving tip: Use dark-hued ketchup for the most lycopene, and squirt on burgers and baked fries or stir with equal parts reduced-fat mayo for a Russian dressing, says Tanya Zuckerbrot, RD, a dietitian in New York City. Or mix with chopped garlic and herbs to marinate grilled chicken, suggests Daniel Stern, executive chef and co-owner of MidAtlantic and R2L restaurants in Philadelphia.

BUCKWHEAT HONEY

Fights aging

Daily dose: 2 to 4 tablespoons

Dark honey like buckwheat or blueberry contains the most antioxidants, say researchers at the University of Illinois Urbana-Champaign, who analyzed 19 varieties. Antioxidants protect cells from the damaging effects of free radicals and may reduce the risk of heart disease, cancer, cognitive decline, and macular degeneration.

Serving tip: Honey has a strong flavor, so add it in small doses to oatmeal, plain yogurt, and tea, and use instead of refined sugar, suggests Stern. Whisk it into homemade salad dressing for a touch of sweetness.

ROSEMARY

Eliminates foodborne carcinogens

Daily dose: 1 to 2 tablespoons

Rosemary minimizes or eliminates carcinogens formed when cooking some foods, say scientists at Kansas State University, who found that seasoning beef with rosemary before grilling can reduce cancer-causing substances called heterocyclic amines by 30 to 100 percent. Danish scientists got similar results when adding rosemary to dough. Acrylamide, a potentially carcinogenic compound, forms in carb-rich foods when heated above 250°F. "By incorporating 1 tablespoon of dried rosemary for each pound of flour, we reduced acrylamide by more than 50 percent," says Leif Skibsted, PhD, a professor of food chemistry at the University of Copenhagen. He believes that the antioxidants in rosemary "scavenge" the harmful compounds.

Serving tip: Add 1 to 2 tablespoons per 2 pounds of pork loin, steak, or lamb, or spread a paste of chopped rosemary, Dijon mustard, garlic, and coarse sea salt on meat before cooking, suggests Marc Meyer, executive chef at Cookshop, Five Points, and Hundred Acres restaurants in New York City. Stuff chicken or turkey with citrus fruit and rosemary sprigs, then roast.

HORSERADISH

Detoxes your body

Daily dose: ¼ teaspoon

Glucosinolates, compounds in the roots and leaves of the horseradish plant, can increase your liver's ability to detoxify carcinogens and may suppress the growth of existing tumors, says a study in the *Journal of Agricultural and Food Chemistry.* Horseradish is one of nature's best sources of glucosinolates. It has up to 10 times more than broccoli, the next-best source.

Serving tip: Mix into ketchup for a cocktail sauce or mustard for a sandwich spread, or add to yogurt to serve with lamb or fish, says Stern. Make a dip, adds Zuckerbrot: Combine 1 cup nonfat Greek yogurt, ½ cup chopped dill, 3 tablespoons bottled horseradish, and ½ teaspoon salt; enjoy with whole wheat pita chips.

OLIVE OIL

Boosts long-term memory

Daily dose: a few tablespoons

Olive oil is a top source of oleic acid, an omega-9 fatty acid that is converted during digestion to oleoylethanolamide (OEA), a hormone that helps keep brain cells healthy. In a new study from the University of California, Irvine, rodents fed OEA were better able to remember how to perform two tasks than those that didn't eat it. Researchers hypothesize that OEA signals the part of the brain responsible for turning short-term memories into long-term ones. "OEA seems to be part of the glue that makes memories stick," says Daniele Piomelli, PhD, a professor of pharmacology and biological chemistry at the university.

Serving tip: Drizzle on roasted veggies or salad, or mix with crushed garlic and a pinch of salt and spread on toasted whole grain bread. Or blend equal parts olive oil, balsamic vinegar, and water with a squeeze of lemon and use as a dip for crisp veggies like radishes or cucumber.

CINNAMON

Stabilizes blood sugar levels

Daily dose: 1 teaspoon

People who added cinnamon—one-half to a heaping teaspoon—to a sweet dish experienced a slower rise in blood sugar than those who didn't consume any, found a series of studies in the *American Journal of Clinical Nutrition*. The spice enhances insulin sensitivity, so it allows you to use more of the glucose in your blood, keeping blood sugar levels stable, says Joanna Hlebowicz, PhD, the studies' lead researcher and a fellow in cardiology at Lund University in Sweden. Adding cinnamon to a carb-heavy or starchy dish may also help stabilize blood sugar after you eat, she adds. Keeping levels stable minimizes sugar highs and lows, and for those with diabetes, it could mean needing less insulin.

Serving tip: Sprinkle on cake, cereal, or a latte. Work into starchy meals, like rice or grain dishes, by grinding together with cumin, coriander, and caraway and adding chopped nuts and dried fruit for a Mediterranean flavor, recommends Meyer.

HOT SAUCE

Curbs appetite

Daily dose: a few dashes

Eating just one meal that contains capsaicin—the compound that gives hot sauce and chile peppers their heat—not only reduces levels of hunger-causing ghrelin but also raises GLP-1, an appetite-suppressing hormone, says new research in the *European Journal of Nutrition.*

Serving tip: Splash on tacos, brown rice, or low-fat tomato or lentil soup. Hot sauce also pairs well with citrus, adds Meyer. Top half a grapefruit with a few shakes plus a teaspoon of brown sugar.

SAUERKRAUT

Eases digestion

Daily dose: $\frac{1}{2}$ cup

Sauerkraut is full of probiotic bacteria such as Lactobacillus plantarum (L. plantarum) that can help relieve the gas, stomach distension, and discomfort associated with irritable bowel syndrome—and may improve the quality of life in up to 95 percent of those with IBS.

Serving tip: Use fresh sauerkraut (it has more probiotic bacteria than jarred varieties) as a relish for grilled meats or lean turkey hot dogs. Or toss into a veggie and tofu stir-fry, says Andrea-Michelle Brekke, RD, a nutritionist in New York City.

CHAPTER 19

HIGH FRUCTOSE CORN SYRUP:
How Dangerous Is It?

An ad campaign attempts to give this sweetener a makeover. We have the full story.

In the grand tradition of nutritional scapegoating, high fructose corn syrup (HFCS) has stepped into the spotlight as dietary enemy number one. It's an easy target. The corn-based sweetener is found throughout the American diet, in everything from sugary foods like soda and cookies to savory products like tomato sauce and salad dressing. That's precisely the problem, say critics who blame the vast quantities we consume for the nation's soaring rates of obesity and diabetes.

But not everyone is convinced. Last June, the Corn Refiners Association launched an ad campaign telling the other side of the story—namely, that HFCS is "made from corn [and] has the same calories as sugar."

The mixed messages have left consumers looking for answers. *Prevention* investigated and found little conclusive evidence to confirm the anti-HFCS crusade. Still, concerned researchers say there are reasons to keep your intake to a minimum. Here we address the most common claims about HFCS and have experts weigh in so you can make the best choice for your health.

"TABLE SUGAR AND HFCS HAVE THE SAME NUMBER OF CALORIES"

The verdict: "Gram for gram, table sugar and high fructose corn syrup are equal in calories," says New York City–based nutritionist Tanya Zuckerbrot, RD. They are also equally sweet. And both consist of two simple sugars—fructose and glucose—in roughly the same proportions (though the two sugars are merely blended together in HFCS, versus chemically bonded in sugar).

Your body breaks down both products in virtually the same way, says Michael F. Jacobson, PhD, with the Center for Science in the Public Interest (CSPI). He adds, "There's no evidence that high fructose corn syrup is worse than sugar once it's in your body."

Still, we know much less about the long-term effects of HFCS than about those of sugar. HFCS was invented in the 1960s and has been used extensively in consumer products since only the late 1970s.

"That's when an increase in the price of sugar helped make less-expensive corn sweeteners more attractive to manufacturers," says Helen H. Jensen, PhD, an agricultural economist at Iowa State University. It may be too soon to say that HFCS and sugar (which has been consumed safely for thousands of years) are the same.

"HFCS IS NATURAL"

The verdict: *Natural* is relative, so think of it this way: HFCS would not exist without the aid of humans. (Of course, neither would table sugar.)

THREE SWEETENERS WITH BONUS BENEFITS

Surprising fact: Some sweeteners do have health benefits. Trade your usual packaged fare for no-added-sugar versions and flavor them with these good-for-you sweeteners. You'll satisfy your sweet tooth, boost your health, and save calories.

ANTIOXIDANT-PACKED SWEETENERS. Molasses, brown sugar, maple syrup, and honey all have intermediate to high levels of the disease-fighting compounds, according to a new *Journal of the American Dietetic Association* study.

SWEET SAVINGS. One packet of maple and brown sugar instant oatmeal has 160 calories; one packet of plain instant oatmeal topped with 1 teaspoon each of maple syrup and brown sugar has 127.

FRESH, FROZEN, OR UNSWEETENED DRIED FRUIT. Research links a diet high in fruit with decreased risk of cardiovascular disease, thanks to its high levels of health-promoting vitamins, minerals, and antioxidants.

SWEET SAVINGS. Six ounces of strawberry fruit-on-the-bottom yogurt packs 170 calories; 6 ounces of nonfat plain Greek yogurt blended with ¼ cup of sliced strawberries has 112.

A DASH OF SPICE. Cloves and cinnamon can lend sweetness to foods while adding minimal calories. A study in the *Journal of Agricultural and Food Chemistry* found that these spices were among the highest in antioxidants out of 30 plants tested.

SWEET SAVINGS. One 16-ounce Cinnamon Dolce Latte from Starbucks has 330 calories; a 16-ounce Caffè Latte topped with cinnamon has 192.

"You don't just squeeze it out of a kernel of corn," explains Dr. Jacobson. The sweetener is made from cornstarch via a process that alters corn's naturally occurring starch molecules. For that reason, Jacobson and CSPI protested an early version of the Corn Refiners Association ads that used the term *natural* in reference to HFCS. Eventually, he says, they took out the word "because it's not natural—it's highly processed."

"HFCS IS RESPONSIBLE FOR THE RISE IN OBESITY IN OUR COUNTRY"

The verdict: Manufacturers started using HFCS in the late '70s, right before America's collective waistline began to expand. Researchers have speculated that the relationship is more than a coincidence. However, a December 2008 supplement to the *American Journal of Clinical Nutrition* found no scientific support for the hypothesis that HFCS is causing obesity in the United States.

Some experts make an indirect case: HFCS, once much cheaper than sugar, cut the cost of sweet, calorie-dense foods, which fueled our sweet tooth—causing weight gain in the process.

"HFCS CONTRIBUTES TO DIABETES RISK"

The verdict: "This notion that high fructose corn syrup is to blame for diabetes isn't exactly accurate," says Zuckerbrot. It probably gained traction alongside the obesity rumor. But we do know that excess calories from any source lead to weight gain, which plays a role in diabetes.

Interestingly, research suggests that a diet high in fructose (the sugar found naturally in fruit) may lead to leptin resistance, a hallmark of diabetes—and thanks to the ubiquity of HFCS, we are getting more fructose in our diets than ever before. Scientists are continuing to explore the possible link.

One clue that there's more to learn: In 2007, researchers at Rutgers University found that sodas sweetened with HFCS have high levels of compounds called reactive carbonyls, which are found in excess in the blood of people with diabetes and may contribute to tissue damage.

"This brings up some interesting concerns, but we don't want to hang our hat on the results of one study," says American Dietetic Association spokesperson Lona Sandon, RD.

Bottom line: More research needs to be done.

"HFCS CONTAINS MERCURY"

The verdict: Nearly half of the 20 HFCS samples tested in a recent study contained small amounts of potentially harmful mercury, according to one report. While the Corn Refiners Association argues that the research was based on outdated information, another study by the Institute for Agriculture and Trade Policy found that one-third of all HFCS-containing foods it bought in the fall of 2008 tested positive for the toxin.

The researchers believe that HFCS is probably the source. A compound known as caustic soda, which is used to separate the corn starch from the kernel, can be tainted with mercury, and there's no way for you to know whether the caustic soda used was contaminated, according to study author David Wallinga, MD, Food and Health Program director at the Institute for Agriculture and Trade Policy. Although much of the US production of caustic soda uses mercury-free technology, not all manufacturers worldwide have followed suit, adding fuel to the argument for minimizing HFCS intake.

"THE FDA SAYS THAT HFCS IS SAFE TO CONSUME, SO IT MUST BE"

The verdict: The FDA has ruled twice that HFCS is "safe" to consume. But the FDA also considers double bacon cheeseburgers safe, and you wouldn't want to eat those every day. Limiting HFCS (and other added sweeteners) does have one well-understood benefit: It will help you lose weight. And that will help prevent disease.

Dr. Jacobson agrees. Although the Corn Refiners Association is successfully pumping up the image of HFCS in the minds of many consumers, he believes that there's more the public should know.

"The ads set the record straight about the similarities between sugar and high fructose corn syrup," he says. "But the responsible message should be 'Consume less of both.'"

SIX FOODS THAT SHOULD NEVER CROSS YOUR LIPS

Clean eating means choosing fruits, vegetables, and meats that are raised, grown, and sold with minimal processing. Often they're organic, and rarely (if ever) should they contain additives. But in some cases, the methods of today's food producers are neither clean nor sustainable. The result is damage to our health, the environment, or both. So we decided to take a fresh look at food through the eyes of the people who spend their lives uncovering what's safe—or not—to eat. We asked them a simple question: "What foods do you avoid?" Their answers don't necessarily make up a "banned foods" list. But reaching for the suggested alternatives might bring you better health—and peace of mind.

The Endocrinologist Won't Eat: Canned Tomatoes

Frederick vom Saal, PhD, is an endocrinologist at the University of Missouri who studies bisphenol A.

THE PROBLEM: The resin linings of tin cans contain bisphenol A, a synthetic estrogen that has been linked to ailments ranging from reproductive problems to heart disease, diabetes, and obesity. Unfortunately, acidity (a prominent characteristic of tomatoes) causes BPA to leach into your food. Studies show that the BPA in most people's bodies exceeds the amount that suppresses sperm production or causes chromosomal damage to the eggs of animals. "You can get 50 micrograms of BPA per liter out of a tomato can, and that's a level that is going to impact people, particularly the young," says Dr. vom Saal. "I won't go near canned tomatoes."

THE SOLUTION: Choose tomatoes in glass bottles (which do not need resin linings), such as the brands Bionaturae and Coluccio. You can also get several types in Tetra Pak boxes, like Trader Joe's and Pomi.

BUDGET TIP: If your recipe allows, substitute bottled pasta sauce for canned tomatoes. Look for pasta sauces with low sodium and few added ingredients, or you may have to adjust the recipe.

The Farmer Won't Eat: Corn-Fed Beef

Joel Salatin is co-owner of Polyface Farms and author of more than half a dozen books on sustainable farming.

THE PROBLEM: Cattle evolved to eat grass, not grains. But farmers today feed their animals corn and soybeans, which fatten up the animals faster for slaughter. More money for cattle farmers (and lower prices at the grocery store) means a lot less nutrition for us. A recent comprehensive study conducted by the USDA and researchers from Clemson University found that compared with corn-fed beef, grass-fed beef is higher in beta-carotene, vitamin E, omega-3s, conjugated linoleic acid (CLA), calcium, magnesium, and potassium; and lower in inflammatory omega-6s and in saturated fats that have been linked to heart disease. "We need to respect the fact that cows are herbivores, and that does not mean feeding them corn and chicken manure," says Salatin.

THE SOLUTION: Buy grass-fed beef, which can be found at specialty grocers, farmers' markets, and nationally at Whole Foods. It's usually labeled because it demands a premium, but if you don't see it, ask your butcher.

BUDGET TIP: Cuts on the bone are cheaper because processors charge extra for deboning. You can also buy direct from a local farmer, which can be as cheap as $5 per pound. To find a farmer near you, search www.eatwild.com.

The Toxicologist Won't Eat: Microwave Popcorn

Olga Naidenko, PhD, is a senior scientist for the Environmental Working Group.

THE PROBLEM: Chemicals, including perfluorooctanoic acid (PFOA), in the lining of the bag are part of a class of compounds that may be linked to infertility in humans, according to a recent study from UCLA. In animal testing, the chemicals cause liver, testicular, and pancreatic cancers. Studies show that microwaving causes the chemicals to vaporize—and migrate into your popcorn. "They stay in your body for years and accumulate there," says Dr. Naidenko, which is why researchers worry that levels in humans could approach the amounts causing cancers in laboratory animals. DuPont and other manufacturers have promised to phase out PFOA by 2015 under a voluntary EPA plan, but millions of bags of popcorn will be sold between now and then.

(continued)

THE SOLUTION: Pop natural kernels the old-fashioned way: in a skillet. For flavorings, you can add real butter or dried seasonings such as dillweed, vegetable flakes, or soup mix.

BUDGET TIP: Popping your own popcorn is dirt cheap.

The Farm Director Won't Eat: Nonorganic Potatoes

Jeffrey Moyer is the chair of the National Organic Standards Board.

THE PROBLEM: Root vegetables absorb herbicides, pesticides, and fungicides that wind up in soil. In the case of potatoes—the nation's most popular vegetable—they're treated with fungicides during the growing season, then sprayed with herbicides to kill off the fibrous vines before harvesting. After they're dug up, the potatoes are treated yet again to prevent them from sprouting. "Try this experiment: Buy a conventional potato in a store, and try to get it to sprout. It won't," says Moyer, who is also farm director of the Rodale Institute (also owned by Rodale Inc., the publisher of *Prevention*). "I've talked with potato growers who say point-blank they would never eat the potatoes they sell. They have separate plots where they grow potatoes for themselves without all the chemicals."

THE SOLUTION: Buy organic potatoes. Washing isn't good enough if you're trying to remove chemicals that have been absorbed into the flesh.

BUDGET TIP: Organic potatoes are only $1 to $2 a pound, slightly more expensive than conventional spuds.

The Fisheries Expert Won't Eat: Farmed Salmon

David Carpenter, MD, director of the Institute for Health and the Environment at the University at Albany, published a major study in the journal *Science* on contamination in fish.

THE PROBLEM: Nature didn't intend for salmon to be crammed into pens and fed soy, poultry litter, and hydrolyzed chicken feathers. As a result, farmed salmon is lower in vitamin D and higher in contaminants, including carcinogens, PCBs, brominated flame retardants, and pesticides such as dioxin and DDT. According to

Dr. Carpenter, the most contaminated fish come from Northern Europe, and they can be found on American menus. "You could eat one of these salmon dinners every 5 months without increasing your risk of cancer," says Dr. Carpenter, whose 2004 fish contamination study got broad media attention. "It's that bad." Preliminary science has also linked DDT to diabetes and obesity, but some nutritionists believe the benefits of omega-3s outweigh the risks. There is also concern about the high level of antibiotics and pesticides used to treat these fish. When you eat farmed salmon, you get dosed with the same drugs and chemicals.

THE SOLUTION: Switch to wild-caught Alaska salmon. If the package says fresh Atlantic, it's farmed. There are no commercial fisheries left for wild Atlantic salmon.

BUDGET TIP: Canned salmon, almost exclusively from wild catch, can be found for as little as $3 a can.

The Cancer Researcher Won't Drink: Milk Produced with Artificial Hormones

Rick North is project director of the Campaign for Safe Food at the Oregon Physicians for Social Responsibility.

THE PROBLEM: Milk producers treat their dairy cattle with recombinant bovine growth hormone (rBGH or rBST, as it is also known) to boost milk production. But rBGH increases udder infections and even pus in the milk. It also leads to higher levels of a hormone called insulin-like growth factor (IGF-1) in milk. In people, high levels of IGF-1 may contribute to breast, prostate, and colon cancers. "When the government approved rBGH, it was thought that IGF-1 from milk would be broken down in the human digestive tract," says North. As it turns out, the casein in milk protects most of it, according to several independent studies. "There's not 100 percent proof that this is increasing cancer in humans," he admits. "However, it's banned in most industrialized countries."

THE SOLUTION: Check labels for rBGH-free, rBST-free, produced without artificial hormones, or organic milk. These phrases indicate rBGH-free products.

BUDGET TIP: Try Walmart's Great Value label, which does not use rBGH.

CHAPTER 20

THE VANISHING Youth Nutrient

Writer Susan Allport unravels why the disappearance of omega-3s from our diet may be responsible for the obesity, heart disease, and cancer epidemics. Oh, and wrinkles, too

When Lisa Kepp* was 2 years old, she was diagnosed with a neurological condition. She had not said a word in her short life—and it wasn't for want of trying. Lisa was so frustrated at not being able to form the words she clearly wanted to say that she flew into temper tantrums 4 or 5 times a day. The family was on pins and needles waiting for the next time the little girl would explode.

A pediatric neurologist diagnosed verbal apraxia, a speech disorder, and recommended that she receive intensive speech therapy. He suggested no other treatment. Lisa's mother had heard, though, about studies linking omega-3 fatty acids to intelligence and healthy brains, and she thought she'd give them a try. She purchased a bottle of Nordic Naturals' Children's DHA in liquid form and began putting half a teaspoon in her daughter's orange juice

*Name has been changed to protect privacy.

233

every morning. Within a week, the young girl was babbling and her tantrums stopped. Amazed, her mother spoke to the doctors, but none of them would engage her, as she puts it, in a conversation about omega-3s. So Lisa continued speech therapy—and her omega-3s—for a year and will be starting preschool this fall with her peers.

A happy anecdote, to be sure. But scientists will admit that without testing, we can't be certain that omega-3s fueled Lisa's recovery. Scientists can, however, point to a growing body of scientific literature that touts the benefits of omega-3 supplementation. Studies show that these special fatty acids accumulate in the brain and can aid children with learning disabilities, reduce violence in prison populations, and even improve everyday mood.

We can only obtain these fats through our diet. They are essential to the development of healthy brains and other metabolically active tissues. Indeed, research from the world's top universities shows that these fats do much more than regulate our brains: They can also lower risk of heart disease, arthritis, and cancer. They even help fight wrinkles and may block fat-cell formation.

How could omega-3s possibly be this powerful? Scientists believe it's because Americans are suffering from a widespread deficiency. A recent study conducted by Dariush Mozaffarian, MD, of the Harvard School of Public Health, found that the absence of these fatty acids in our diet is responsible annually for up to 96,000 premature deaths in this country. Scientists, however,

→ PREVENTION Alert!

BEEF UP YOUR HEALTHY FAT INTAKE

Americans are eating too few heart-healthy omega-3 fatty acids and too many inflammation-promoting omega-6s. And now data from a massive Chinese study finds that women who eat the most omega-6s and the fewest omega-3s have nearly double the risk of colorectal cancer, compared with those who consume the opposite. For the healthiest ratio, eat fewer processed foods, in which omega-6s are abundant, and more natural sources of omega-3s, such as leafy greens, grass-fed beef, and fatty fish.

THREE EASY WAYS TO INCREASE OMEGA-3S

The competition between omega-3s and omega-6s is happening all the time, not just when we take our fish oil capsules. The best way to ensure you have a healthy balance of essential fats is to have a source of omega-3s—and not too many omega-6s—at every meal.

EAT MORE GREENS. Leafy greens, legumes, and potatoes have a better balance of omega-3s to omega-6s than most seeds and grains. Omega-3s live in leaves as the omega-3 ALA (alpha-linolenic acid). Animals (like us) convert ALA into even more dynamic omega-3s: EPA and DHA. This conversion is somewhat inefficient, however, and that's why the next steps are so important.

EAT HEALTHIER MEATS. Cows raised on grass produce meat, milk, and cheese with many more omega-3s than their corn-and-soy-fed counterparts. Chickens fed a diet rich in flax and greens produce eggs that are as high in EPA and DHA as many species of fish. Some would argue that grass-fed meats are more expensive than grain-fed, but the former come without the very steep medical price tag of a diet high in omega-6s.

EAT FISH. Fish can also be a sustainable part of our new diet, as moderate fish consumption will be more effective when our diet has fewer omega-6s. Try to eat at least two meals of fish per week. Fish oil supplements can also help, as Lisa's mother found, though they're not a long-term solution to this widespread nutritional deficiency.

are learning that fixing this nutritional deficiency is a bit more complicated than simply telling people to eat more fish.

OUR COLLECTIVE OMEGA-3 DEFICIENCY . . .

Every once in a while, a discovery comes along that changes everything about the way we see the world. In the early 16th century, Nicolaus Copernicus had such a moment when he discovered that Earth was not the center of the universe. Our new understanding of essential fats is that kind of discovery, and I was lucky enough, as a science writer, to make a small yet key contribution. While researching a book on omega-3s, I realized that the essential fats—the omega-3s and their close cousins, the omega-6s—change with the seasons. It might sound like a small idea, but it may soon fundamentally change the way you think about food.

First, let's start with omega-3s, what I'll call the spring fats. These are likely the most abundant fats in the world, but they don't originate in fish, as many believe. Rather, they are found in the green leaves of plants. Fish are full of omega-3s because they eat phytoplankton (the microscopic green plants of the ocean) and seaweed. In plants, these special fatty acids help turn sunlight into sugars, the basis of life on Earth. The spring fats speed up metabolism. They are fats that animals (humans included) use to get ready for times of activity, like the mating season. They're found in the highest concentrations in all the most active tissues: brains, eyes, hearts, the tails of sperm, the flight muscles of hummingbirds. Because fish have so many of these fats in their diets, they can be active in cold, dark waters. These fats protect our brains from neurological disorders and enable our hearts to beat billions of times without incident. But they are vanishing from our diet, and you'll soon understand why.

PREVENTION Alert!

OMEGAS IN A GLASS

A daily serving of red wine may boost the effects of heart-healthy omega-3 fatty acids, reports new research. Women ages 26 to 65 who drank one glass daily had higher blood levels of omega-3s—regardless of their fish consumption (the nutrient's top source). Scientists say that the polyphenols in wine may alter the metabolism of omega-3s. One caution: Women with a family history of breast cancer should get omega-3s from fish, as studies show that even one daily drink may increase risk of the disease.

. . . AND OUR OMEGA-6 SURPLUS

Next up are the omega-6s, what I'll call the fall fats. They originate in plants as well, but in the seeds of plants rather than the leaves. The fall fats are simply storage fats for plants. Animals require both—omega-3s and omega-6s—in their diets and their tissues. But omega-6s are slower and stiffer than omega-3s. Plus, they promote blood clotting and inflammation, the underlying causes of many diseases, including heart disease and arthritis. Omega-3s, on the other hand, promote blood flow and very little inflammation, which may prevent things like heart disease. The proper mix of these two fats helps create tissue with the right amount of blood flow and inflammation. But because they're in constant competition to enter our cells, if your diet consists of too many omega-6s, your body will be deficient in omega-3s. And that is what's been happening to us as we've been eating more and more seed fats in the form of soybean, corn, and other vegetable oils.

Since 1909, according to the USDA, Americans have more than doubled their daily intake of omega-6s—from about 7 grams to around 18. One hundred years ago, heart disease was much less common in this country. Over the past century, though, heart disease has risen in tandem with our increasing intake of these seed fats, or omega-6s, according to the American Heart Association (AHA). So have neurological disorders like Lisa's, as well as depression, arthritis, obesity, insulin resistance, and many cancers. While other dietary factors such as increased consumption of calories, trans fats, and sugar undoubtedly contributed, our essential fatty acid imbalance is a key player in most of these illnesses.

Over the same time period, omega-3s began disappearing from our food supply. Cows used to be raised on grass and other greens, producing meat, milk, and cheese with much higher concentrations of omega-3s. These were the animal products that our grandparents and great-grandparents grew up on, before industrial feedlots replaced family farms. Now these livestock are fed corn and soy, and their tissues are swamped with omega-6s. Chickens, too, used to eat grass and grass-eating bugs. Those chickens produced eggs and meat that were high in omega-3s, but now they're fed full of omega-6-rich fall fats.

ONE TIME TO SKIP SUPPLEMENTS

More than 50 percent of people take natural remedies—such as fish oil, echinacea, ginseng, garlic, and ginkgo—before surgery, but only 30 to 60 percent tell their doctors. These remedies and others can cause bleeding, heart attack, stroke, allergic reactions, and inadequate sedation when mixed with anesthetic and anticoagulant drugs. As part of your presurgical prep, mention any supplements you take. You may be advised to stop for 3 weeks before your procedure.

We are now eating a diet that is supposed to fatten us up for winter, when weather is harsh and calories are scarce. But today food is never scarce for the average American. The base of our food supply has shifted from leaves to seeds, and this simple change means our bodies are storing more fat, leading to obesity and all its associated diseases.

HOW WE GOT HERE

This is all too simple to be true, you might say. But arriving at this understanding was anything but simple. In the 1930s, the first family of essential fats was discovered and mapped by George and Mildred Burr at the University of Minnesota. These were the omega-6s. It was another 40 years before omega-3s were also found to be essential, by a researcher at the Hormel Institute named Ralph Holman. A great deal happened to our food supply in those decades. Due to farm subsidies, the acres of soybeans, for example, grown in the United States exploded from about 4 million to 70 million. Oil processors like Archer Daniels Midland mastered the process of extracting oil from these and other seeds, and vegetable seed oils—thought to be healthy—began to dominate our food supply as they were added to the foods that make up the center aisles of the grocery store.

At the same time, food chemists discovered that rancidity in packaged foods was caused by the oxidation of some minor but pesky fats: omega-3s. Scientists extended the shelf life of processed foods such as cookies, chips, cakes, breads,

10 EASY WAYS TO REDUCE OMEGA-6s

Very simply, we must decrease our consumption of omega-6 oils. Snacking on seeds, edamame, and whole foods is still healthy. But cut back on processed foods, which are high in omega-6-laden seed oils. At home, cook with oils and fats with a healthy balance of omega-6s to omega-3s. A few oil seeds—canola and flax, for instance—have a very favorable ratio of the two families of essential fats, and they can be used by themselves (canola) or in combination with other oils (flax) to change the balance of omega-3s to omega-6s. Mix flax and canola with any of the other seed oils such as corn and safflower, to produce a healthy blend. If you're curious about olive oil, it's still fine to use, as it's not high in omega-3 or omega-6s; it's fairly neutral. Here are some other simple steps.

1. Replace processed cereal with cereal or oatmeal that contains flaxseed.
2. Make your own salad dressing with a mix of canola and olive oil.
3. Eat less fast food because it's all very high in omega-6 seed oils.
4. Look for potato chips that are fried in canola oil rather than cottonseed, soy, safflower, or sunflower oil.
5. Substitute walnuts for other nuts when you can because they're a seed that's high in omega-3s.
6. Make your own baked goods, replacing half the butter with canola oil.
7. Check food labels to avoid hydrogenated and partially hydrogenated oils.
8. Avoid omega supplements that contain both omega-3s and omega-6s. You'll see these labeled with terms like Complete Omega.
9. Choose grass-fed pork, chicken, beef, or bison whenever you can.
10. Avoid farmed fish because they are often fed corn and soy.

and spreads by removing omega-3s—a nutrient that no one thought mattered. Health agencies, like the AHA, and the US government also promoted omega-6s, because seed oils are low in saturated fat and free of cholesterol. So omega-6 oils, such as corn and soybean, they thought, were good for the heart.

Scientists have known since the early 1970s, however, that omega-6s also promote blood clotting and inflammation, two immediate and direct causes of heart disease. But because omega-6s were essential, doctors thought you had to take the good with the bad. By the time they learned that omega-3s protect our hearts and fight inflammation, omega-6s were already the foundation of our modern food supply.

Then, in the 1980s, epidemiological studies published in prestigious journals like the *New England Journal of Medicine* showed that fish-eating populations in Greenland and Japan are much less prone to heart disease. Omega-3s became associated with fish (rather than with green leaves), and that became the method recommended by such organizations as the AHA for us to obtain our omega-3s. The only problem is that eating more fish isn't a sustainable solution, as many of the world's fisheries are at the brink of collapse, according to a major study recently published in *Science.* Literally, there aren't enough fish in the world's oceans.

OBESITY'S REAL CAUSE?

It wasn't until Australian researchers showed a clear difference between membranes full of omega-3 fats and ones full of omega-6 fats—a clear metabolic difference—that I explored the seasonal aspects of these two fats. When Tony Hulbert, PhD, at Australia's University of Wollongong, determined that the metabolism of a species—every species on the planet—is a function of the amount of omega-3s in its tissues, I began to connect the dots.

It is probably no coincidence, I realized, as I researched my book *The Queen of Fats,* that leaves are the most metabolically active tissues in plants, and brains and eyes are the most metabolically active tissues in animals: They are both full of omega-3 fats. Omega-3s speed up the activity of cells.

It is no coincidence, I realized, that omega-6s are simply a storage fat for plants. Both omega-6s and omega-3s play many vital, essential roles in animals, as I cannot emphasize enough. But in plants, the only role of omega-6s is to serve as a storage fat. Omega-6s are also the main polyunsaturated fat in the storage fat of animals: white adipose tissue—the belly fat of every overweight American.

It is no coincidence that hibernating animals such as the yellow-bellied marmot of Colorado do not go into hibernation when their diet is full of omega-3s, as it is in the spring and summer. Their diet must change to one rich in omega-6 seeds before these animals will slow down for the winter.

It is no coincidence that animals that migrate long distances—like the semipalmated sandpiper, which flies from Nova Scotia to South America—fill up on omega-3s for their long journey. These birds know what human athletes are just starting to learn: High omega-3 concentrations in muscle membranes lead to improved performance.

So it is no coincidence that as America shifted its diet—from one based on green leaves to one based on seeds—we became fatter and fatter and sicker and sicker. Our hibernation diet is exposing us to epidemics of obesity, diabetes, heart disease, cancer, and brain disorders. Even infants, according to the Child & Family Research Institute of the University of British Columbia, are getting fatter—long before they could ever be accused of overeating—when they are fed formulas high in omega-6s. Sure, America's seed-based foods are remarkably cheap, but we spend the lowest percentage of our income on food and more on health care than any other country in the world.

Since publishing *The Queen of Fats,* I've continued to comb the literature for studies that shed light on the role that the essential fats play in nature. I came across one not too long ago in the journal *Lipids* about the African kudu and impala, showing that these animals also experience a shift in the amounts of omega-3s and omega-6s in their diets over the course of the rainy and dry seasons—rather than our seasons based on day length. It made me realize that these shifts are universal signals, experienced and interpreted by animals all over the planet—at least until we humans came along and devised a way of eating a diet rich in seed fats all year long.

There's a solution to our imbalance, but change is difficult, and we must first accept that polyunsaturates—omega-3s and omega-6s—are not one big happy family; rather, they are two competing families—spring fats and fall fats—with very different effects on cells and health. Once we've accepted that, making the necessary dietary improvements is relatively easy.

CHAPTER 21

NUTRIENTS
Even Healthy Women Miss

These vitamins and minerals have surprising essential benefits. Here's how to ensure you're getting them all.

Quick: Did you get enough vitamin E today? Even if you're diligent about your diet, you're likely to fall short on this and four other critical nutrients, according to recent USDA figures on the average amounts most midlife women consume. And with headlines questioning the value of multivitamins, it's even more important to make up the difference with tasty, readily available foods, says Lisa Hark, PhD, RD, a Philadelphia-based family-nutrition expert.

Simple changes to your diet can provide a powerful defense against disease. "With food, you're getting not just isolated nutrients, as you might in a supplement, but a full range of them in the form nature intended," says Dr. Hark, coauthor of *Nutrition for Life*.

Here is where you may fall short—and how to measure up.

VITAMIN E

You need: 15 milligrams per day

You probably get: 6.4 milligrams per day

Your shortfall: 57 percent

This powerful antioxidant protects your cells, helps them to communicate with each other, and defends your skin against UV damage. If you don't get enough vitamin E, you may have problems absorbing other nutrients.

Help make it up: Choose two or three daily.

- ¼ cup dry roasted sunflower seeds: Eat out of hand or toss on salads.
- ¼ cup wheat germ: Sprinkle these flakes into yogurt.
- 1 tablespoon vegetable oil: Use instead of butter to sauté kale, Swiss chard, or other E-rich leafy greens.
- 1 cup red bell pepper: Chop and simmer in pasta sauce.
- 1 cup low-sodium canned white beans: Mash with spices, and use as a dip with celery sticks.

POTASSIUM

You need: 4,700 milligrams per day

You probably get: 2,458 milligrams per day

Your shortfall: 48 percent

This electrolyte keeps your nervous system humming and your muscles toned. It also helps keep your blood pressure at normal levels. If you don't get enough, you may feel irritable, weak, and fatigued. To avoid this, you must eat enough potassium-rich foods and control sodium. That's because the two minerals need to be balanced in your body, and either too little potassium or too much sodium (which is often found in excess in packaged foods) can cause problems.

Help make it up: Pick three or four daily.

- 1 medium baked potato, skin on: Top with salsa or chopped chives for a low-fat side dish.
- 1 cup edamame: Steam with snow peas and corn kernels; let cool slightly, and then toss with dressing for a quick warm salad.
- 1 cup cooked spinach: Incorporate into a pasta dish.
- 1 cup cooked lentils: Have a bowl of low-sodium lentil soup.
- 1 cup sliced banana: Use a blender to whir into smoothies.

CALCIUM

You need: 1,000 to 1,200 milligrams per day

You probably get: 800 milligrams per day

Your shortfall: 20 to 33 percent

This mighty mineral builds strong bones, and that means a lower risk of osteoporosis for you. Calcium can help prevent some other major diseases as well. In a study of nearly 84,000 women by Tufts-New England Medical Center, scientists found that those who consumed at least 1,200 milligrams of calcium daily (along with at least 800 IU of vitamin D, which helps absorption of the mineral) had a 33 percent lower risk of developing type 2 diabetes.

Help make it up: Choose three or four daily.

- 8 ounces low-fat plain yogurt: For dessert, pair with fresh or thawed frozen berries and garnish with mint.
- 3 ounces canned sardines with bones: Quarter the sardines while they're still in the can. Toss with chopped fresh tomatoes and salad dressing, and serve over mesclun mix.
- 1 ounce low-fat cheese: Grate reduced-fat Parmesan into risotto, or use to top pasta.
- ½ cup tofu: Stir-fry with veggies.
- 1 cup cooked chopped bok choy: Warm in broth for a calcium-rich soup.

VITAMIN A

You need: 700 micrograms per day

You probably get: 558 micrograms per day

Your shortfall: 20 percent

This nutrient powers your eyesight, especially your night vision, and keeps your skin, gums, and teeth healthy. It also boosts your immune system and helps you fight off viruses. The older you get, the more you seem to require it to protect cognitive function. A study at Utah State University found that older adults with high intakes of antioxidants, including carotene (from which your body makes vitamin A), had a slower rate of mental decline.

Help make it up: Have one or two daily.

- 1 small sweet potato: Baked, it's a flavorful, brightly hued side dish.
- ¼ cup canned pumpkin: Use along with a dash of cinnamon to jazz up whole wheat pancake batter.
- 10 medium baby carrots: Use as dippers for hummus.
- 1 cup cantaloupe cubes: Dollop with reduced-fat cottage cheese, and drizzle with honey.
- ½ cup dried apricots: Chop and sprinkle on muesli.

MAGNESIUM

You need: 320 milligrams per day

You probably get: 267 milligrams per day

Your shortfall: 17 percent

Magnesium is used in hundreds of chemical activities in the body, ranging from storing energy to helping your genes function properly. It keeps your nerves and muscles toned, your bones strong, and your blood circulating steadily. This mineral is so influential that women who got at least the recommended amount cut their risk of metabolic syndrome by 38 percent or more, reported a study by the Centers for Disease Control. The serious, increasingly common syndrome, affecting some 50 million Americans, is a constellation of risk factors for heart disease and diabetes that includes excess abdominal fat, high blood pressure, and more.

Help make it up: Get three or four daily.

- 1 cup cooked black beans: Toss into a salad, along with chopped cilantro.
- 1 ounce (6 to 8 whole) Brazil nuts: Chop and sprinkle on breakfast cereal.
- 1 cup okra: Simmer fresh or frozen chopped okra in chicken soup or stew.
- 1 cup cooked brown rice: Use as an accompaniment to stir-fry.
- 1 ounce almonds: Toast slivered almonds for a minute in a skillet over low heat, then sprinkle on fruit salad.

CHAPTER 22

THE SUPERBUG
in Your Supermarket

A potentially deadly new strain of antibiotic-resistant microbes may be widespread in our food supply. Protect your loved ones with Prevention's *Special Report.*

About 2 years ago, dozens of workers at a large chicken hatchery in Arkansas began experiencing mysterious skin rashes, with painful lumps scattered over their hands, arms, and legs.

"They hurt real bad," says Joyce Long, 48, a 32-year veteran of the hatchery where, until recently, workers handled eggs and chicks with bare hands. "When we went and got cultured, doctors told us we had a superbug." Its name, she learned, was MRSA, or methicillin-resistant Staphylococcus aureus. This form of staph bacteria developed a mutation that resists antibiotics (including methicillin), making it hard to treat, even lethal. According to the CDC, certain types of MRSA infections kill 18,000 Americans a year—more than die from AIDS.

Soon co-workers at the nearby processing plant, where hundreds of thousands of chicken carcasses are prepped daily for sale, began finding the lumps. Dean Reeves, 50, an 11-year employee, went to the hospital with an excruciating bump on her thigh that she thought was a spider bite. It wasn't: She, too, had contracted MRSA, as had her husband, Bill, 46, who also works at the facility. Since late 2007, Dean has had monthly relapses. Even the safety glasses, gloves, and smocks workers wear (along with upgraded regular cleaning of equipment) aren't enough to protect them, says Bill.

"We work so fast, we often stick ourselves with knives or scissors and get blood on us from head to foot." When a swelling rose over one of his eyes, he was told he might go blind; if the infection progressed to his brain, he'd die.

Did any food safety agency test for MRSA in this plant's chickens, which were then sold to the public and served on American dinner tables? Did any government organization determine the source of the outbreak? Calls to the USDA, CDC, and Arkansas Department of Health yielded a no to both questions. The poultry company that owns the operation did not respond to multiple requests for a comment from *Prevention*. Yet in recent years, studies have found MRSA in retail cuts of pork, chicken, beef, and other meats in the United States, Europe, and Asia.

To get answers, we investigated how MRSA has entered our food supply with limited government response; we considered the massive use of antibiotics in agriculture and its role in creating resistant microbes like MRSA; and we examined the safety of supermarket meat. Here, we offer our findings and expert advice to protect you and your family.

ARE YOU AT RISK?

You've probably heard of people contracting certain strains of MRSA in hospitals, where it causes many illnesses: postsurgical infections, pneumonia, bacteremia, and more. Others encounter different types of the bug in community centers such as gyms, where skin contact occurs and items like sports equipment are shared; this form causes skin infections that may become systemic and turn lethal.

Then in 2008, a new source and strain of MRSA emerged in the United States. Researcher Tara Smith, PhD, an assistant professor of epidemiology at the University of Iowa, studied two large Midwestern hog farms and found the strain, ST398, in 45 percent of farmers and 49 percent of pigs. The startling discovery—and the close connection between animal health and our own that it implied—caused widespread publicity and much official hand-wringing. To date, though, the government has yet to put a comprehensive MRSA inspection process in place, let alone fix our problematic meat-production system.

You might not have the same close contact with meat that a processing plant worker has, but scientists warn there is reason for concern: Most of us handle meat daily, as we bread chicken cutlets, trim fat from pork, or form chopped beef into burgers. Cooking does kill the microbe, but MRSA thrives on skin, so you can contract it by touching infected raw meat when you have a cut on your hand, explains Stuart Levy, MD, a Tufts University professor of microbiology and medicine. MRSA also flourishes in nasal passages, so touching your nose after touching meat gives the bug another way into your body, adds Dr. Smith.

TAINTED MEAT EXPOSED

Extensive research in Europe and Asia has found MRSA in many food animal species, and in the past year, US researchers have begun testing meat sold here. Scientists at Louisiana State University Agricultural Center tested 120 cuts of locally purchased meat and found MRSA in 4 percent of the pork and 1 percent of the beef. A University of Maryland scientist found it in 1 out of 300 pork samples from the Washington, DC, area. And a study in Canada (from which we import thousands of tons of meat annually) found MRSA in 9 percent of 212 pork samples. The percentages may be small, but according to the USDA, Americans eat more than 180 million pounds of meat every day.

"When you consider the tiny size of the meat studies, the fact that they found any contamination at all is amazing," says Steven Roach, public health program director for Food Animal Concerns Trust.

In some cases, the tainted meat probably came from infected animals; in others, already infected humans could have passed on MRSA to the meat during processing. Regardless of where it originated, even a small proportion of contaminated meat could mean a tremendous amount of MRSA out there.

"We need more US research to figure out what's going on," says Roach.

MRSA is so common in the United States that it accounts for more than half of all soft-tissue and skin infections in ERs. The CDC estimates that invasive MRSA infections (those that entered the bloodstream) number more than 94,000 a year. Even more troubling, if you add up the other types of illnesses MRSA can cause, including urinary tract infections, pneumonia, and inpatient skin infections, the total could be 8 to 11 times more than that, reports a study by epidemiologist William Jarvis, MD, of the Association for Professionals in Infection Control and Epidemiology. The numbers are high and rising: From 1996 to 2005, MRSA-related hospitalizations increased nearly tenfold.

People who get MRSA need ever more powerful medication. "Staph-related infections have become serious illnesses that can require hospitalization and stronger drugs," says Georges C. Benjamin, MD, executive director of the American Public Health Association (APHA). For hatchery worker Long, doctors went through several antibiotics, with little success. The swellings would subside, then reappear. "Every time I went back to work, I got it again, for a total of 10 times," she says.

ANIMAL PHARM

Scientists know that antibiotic overuse in humans caused ordinary staph to become resistant, says Dr. Levy. And they know the large amounts of meds used by agriculture caused other bacteria, such as E. coli and Salmonella, to develop resistance.

"Now we're looking at the relationship between antibiotic use on farms and MRSA," he says.

It's an important mission, as industrial agriculture is the country's largest antibiotic user: Animals consume nearly 70 percent of these meds, perhaps more than 24 million pounds a year, says the Union of Concerned Scientists. The drugs compensate for the often unsanitary conditions in the country's

HOW TO STAY SAFE

Experts suggest using the following tips to help reduce your risk of exposure to MRSA in meats.

Shop Smarter

Look for the USDA organic seal. Organic meat might be less likely to have antibiotic-resistant or disease-causing organisms, as the animal hasn't been fed antibiotics, hormones to promote growth, or animal by-products. Other labels, such as "no antibiotics added," are not verified by independent testing.

Log on to www.eatwellguide.org to search for listings of stores and restaurants that offer no-antibiotic-use, grass-fed, or organic meats.

Stock up on nonmeat protein sources such as beans, lentils, and tofu and swap them in for meat now and then. Visit www.prevention.com/veggies for recipe ideas.

Cook Safer

Wash your hands with hot, soapy water before and after you prep meat. Never touch raw meat and then your nose, as MRSA thrives on skin and in nasal passages.

Keep scrapes and cuts covered with waterproof bandages or use rubber gloves. MRSA and other pathogens can use the openings as entry points.

Clean cutting boards and utensils that come in contact with meat with hot, soapy water to avoid cross-contamination.

Make it well-done to kill MRSA and other foodborne bacteria: For pork and beef, the internal temp should be 170°F; for chicken, 165°F.

For more safety tips and guidelines, visit www.prevention.com/links.

19,000 factory farms—also called concentrated animal feeding operations, or CAFOs—where about half our meat is produced. Long gone are many family farms with animals grazing on pastureland, says Robert Martin, senior officer of the Pew Environment Group.

"Instead, they're packed into cramped quarters, never going outdoors, living in their waste," he says. A swine CAFO may house thousands of hogs; a poultry operation, hundreds of thousands of chickens. "As a result, you need to suppress infection."

The large amounts of antibiotics used in CAFOs include drugs critical to curing human illnesses, he says. Premixed animal feed can contain medications you may have taken, such as tetracycline and cephalosporin (Keflex is a familiar brand). You can also buy a 50-pound bag of antibiotics at a feed store to add to your animals' chow—no prescription necessary, confirms Amy Meyer, communications and outreach coordinator for the Missouri Farmers Union.

Most of the antibiotics given to CAFO animals are used not only to fight infection, but also to stimulate growth, says David Wallinga, MD, Food and Health Program director at the Institute for Agriculture and Trade Policy. The near constant exposure to less-than-therapeutic levels of antibiotics allows the resistant bacteria to survive; they can then be transferred to people, he says. This needless use of medication is what doctors try to avoid when they don't prescribe antibiotics for a simple cold.

"These operations are reservoirs of antibiotic resistance," says Dr. Smith.

In the areas surrounding CAFOs, docs see firsthand how MRSA impacts the community. Phillip McClure, DO, practices in Trenton, Missouri, which is home to many hog farms. MRSA infections have risen as the number of pigs has grown, he says. "Both CAFO workers and others get them," says Dr. McClure, who treats an MRSA-related skin problem every month. That may be because you can pick up MRSA and not show symptoms for years. Meanwhile, you can pass it to others by doing something as simple as sharing a towel. Kim Howland, 44, a former hog CAFO worker in Oklahoma, fears she did just that, when in 2007, her husband and daughter developed MRSA skin infections.

"My co-workers told me about lumps they had, and I realized I could have become a carrier," she says. Howland, who left her job, wasn't tested at the time, so she'll never know if she gave MRSA to her family.

Concerned about the risks of CAFOs (including increased antibiotic resistance, pollution, and disease in nearby areas), the APHA back in 2003 called for a moratorium on building new ones.

FOUR-STAR FOOD SAFETY

Here's how professional chefs dodge kitchen dangers daily, from foodborne illness to cuts and burns.

"The sink is often the dirtiest place in the kitchen, so never place food directly in it. Use a colander to wash fruit or veggies."—Donna Mintz, owner, Basil & Barbells in New York

"Always wear plastic kitchen gloves when handling chile peppers. They'll protect your eyes and skin and prevent transfer of the pungent taste and smell to other foods."—James Muir, executive chef, Rosa Mexicano in Washington, DC

"Keep your knives sharp. Dull ones are more likely to slip and cause accidents."—Marc Collins, executive chef, Circa 1886 at the Wentworth Mansion in Charleston, South Carolina

"Prevent contamination by using one hand to handle raw meat and poultry and the other to reach into containers."—Joel Hough, chef de cuisine, Cookshop in New York

"Fill up a food processor or blender only halfway to avoid spills. Heat can expand the volume of soups and sauces."—Philippe Bertineau, head chef at Balthazar in New York

"Keep a spray bottle of water-bleach solution (one full cap per quart of water) handy to sanitize plastic cutting boards between tasks."—David Kamen, professor, Culinary Institute of America

"Keep your most perishable items toward the back of the refrigerator, where it's consistently cool—unlike the fridge door."—Dave Lieberman, chef, the Food Network

WHO'S WATCHING OUT FOR YOU?

Until recently, the CDC has acknowledged the presence of MRSA in meat but downplayed the danger. In 2008, then CDC director Julie Louise Gerberding, MD, MPH, wrote that foodborne transmission of MRSA is "possible" but, if it happens, "likely accounts for a very small proportion of human infections in the US." Liz Wagstrom, DVM, assistant vice president of science and technology for the National Pork Board, agrees, saying that this kind of transmission would be extremely rare. Neither group could provide an estimate when queried by *Prevention*, but considering the high numbers of MRSA infections, even a tiny percentage could be a lot of people.

One reason the CDC and the National Pork Board must guess about transmission rates—and why we don't know exactly how many MRSA-related infections occur—is that the federal government doesn't collect data on MRSA outbreaks, says Karen Steuer, director of government relations for the Pew Environment Group. According to the US Government Accountability Office, there's no testing for MRSA on farms. And the National Antimicrobial Resistance Monitoring System tests just 400 retail cuts of meat each month for four drug-resistant bacteria—which don't include MRSA.

"These gaps in data keep us in the dark," says Steuer. Without farm-to-fork surveillance, it's difficult to connect problems at a certain farm to MRSA outbreaks. "If we don't fix this, mortality rates will go much higher," she says. "We have an impending crisis."

A rising tide of concern is firing up health care activists and congressional policy makers to contain the MRSA threat. Several ideas are on the government's table. Keep Antibiotics Working, a national coalition of health and science organizations, calls for more federal research on MRSA and meat. In Congress, Representative Rosa L. DeLauro suggests giving all supervision of food—now split among many agencies—to just one, which may improve oversight. And Representative Louise Slaughter, MSPH, reportedly Congress's only microbiologist, wants to trim agriculture's use of antibiotics to only those drugs that are not essential for human use. In 2009, she reintroduced the Preservation of Antibiotics for Medical Treatment Act, and the late Senator Edward Kennedy submitted a related bill in the Senate.

Bottom line, says Roach, we need to think of ways to raise animals that prevent them from getting sick in the first place. And we must move quickly, adds Slaughter: "As a scientist and mother, I cannot overstate the urgency. We should be able to buy food without worrying about exposing our family to potentially deadly bacteria that no longer responds to medical treatment."

"I'M HEALTHIER THAN EVER AT 46!"

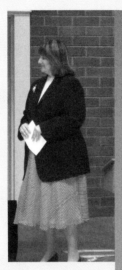
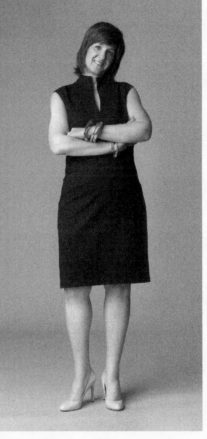

Giving birth to my daughter motivated me to take control of my health and start eating smart.

by Debra Lambert

I was 43 years old and pregnant with my first child, but what should have been the happiest time of my life was one of the scariest. At the beginning of my pregnancy, I weighed more than 200 pounds and was quickly gaining. I developed gestational diabetes, and if I didn't get it under control, I could put my baby at risk for obesity and type 2 diabetes. I didn't want her to have to struggle with weight like I did.

This was the wake-up call that I needed. I met with a dietitian and took control of my blood sugar. The gestational diabetes was gone as soon as I delivered my beautiful baby, but I was almost 280 pounds and at risk for type 2 diabetes. I knew I had to make a change if I wanted to see my daughter graduate from college.

Prevention Intervention

By the time Madelyn was 2, I had shed the 60 pounds I gained during my pregnancy. But at 216 pounds, I was determined to slim down and get healthy once and for all. That's when I read about the *Flat Belly Diet.* Women lost weight adding dark chocolate and nuts to a well-balanced meal? Where do I sign up?

I bought the book, and it didn't take me long to realize that fresh, healthy food was even tastier than the junk of my pre-pregnancy days. Eating four 400-calorie meals daily left me feeling satisfied. And when I needed motivation, I turned to www.flatbellydiet.com; it connected me with people experiencing the same thing I was.

A Lotta Help from My Friends

Almost daily, I was on the message boards, getting advice from other dieters. My first week I was completely overwhelmed, but then someone on the boards said, "Take a deep breath. Just do what you can, and it will be good enough." That's exactly what I needed to hear. Week after week, the pounds kept dropping. But the best part is that I'm teaching my daughter about good nutrition. I'm still active on the site, but these days I'm the one encouraging others. The only thing better than losing the weight is knowing I'm helping others do the same.

Here are my top tips.

Pick a realistic diet plan. I tried other diets where I ate less than 1,200 calories daily, but I couldn't keep up with them. This one was the perfect fit!

Prepare to succeed. Every night I planned and assembled my meals for the following day. In the morning, I just had to grab them and go—no prep work to slow me down.

Measure everything! When you're trying to lose weight, every calorie counts. Stick to correct portions or you could stall your weight loss.

See beyond the scale. Relish small signs that the diet is working. Is it easier to cross your legs? Are your rings fitting better?

Embrace mini challenges. I used to avoid working out, but on the diet I had much more energy. I started walking and realized exercising was easy. I just ran my first 5-K race!

Part5

MIND
MATTERS

CHAPTER 23

HOME
Healing

Soothe your senses and heal stress with easy, cheap home improvements. Science now reveals how these simple steps relax and rejuvenate.

Your living space should serve as a relaxing retreat from the stress of everyday life. Indeed, a growing body of research called "sensory science" supports the notion of home as a sanctuary. Experts have found that the environment you create has a big impact on your outlook and sense of well-being.

"Everything from the pictures on the wall to the slipcover on your couch can have a positive influence on your mood and attitude," says environmental psychologist Sally Augustin, PhD, president of the design firm PlaceCoach in Los Angeles. Make the following small changes to nourish your senses and turn your home into a healing haven.

TOUCH: COZY FABRICS

Textile researchers have found that holding certain types of cloth can evoke powerful emotions. When female students evaluated 10 different fabrics in one British study, both corduroy and fleece elicited feelings of contentment.

Try: Buying a corduroy slipcover for your couch, or draping a fleece throw over the back of a sofa or chair. If you're in the market for new furniture, look for "stain repellent" and "water-resistant" on the label. Newer fabrics with this designation likely have a microscopic "peach fuzz" that makes them feel plush even as it wards off stains, says Maureen S. MacGillivray, PhD, a professor of apparel and textiles at Central Michigan University.

SEE: CLEAN SURFACES

Clutter isn't just unpleasant to look at, it can also be distressing—especially when you don't have control over it. In one study at Washington State University, volunteers looked at photographs of offices in various states of disarray. The bigger the mess, the more anxious people felt, even though their own offices were just as disorganized.

Try: Aiming your sights on the kitchen counter, which is a prime dumping spot. Place a basket for mail next to your phone; banish hats, gloves, and sunglasses to a bin underneath the counter so it's out of sight but still within reach. And every day, spend a little time tidying up. Because cleaning is a physical activity, it further provides a mood lift: Last year, researchers found that people who did 20 minutes of housework suffered from less anxiety and depression.

BREATHE: FLORAL AND FOOD SCENTS

In a Rutgers University study, women who received bouquets reported positive feelings even a few days later. Researchers speculate that flowers contain certain compounds that improve well-being.

Try: Scattering jasmine and hyacinth around the house. These blossoms boosted mood and lowered anxiety levels in studies. Cinnamon and peppermint are two other aromas proven to perk you up. To scent your home naturally, use an essential-oil diffuser or place cinnamon sticks in table centerpieces.

HEAR: PLEASANT SOUNDS

Cornell University researchers found that even low-level noise—like the sound of someone typing—might ramp up levels of the stress hormone epinephrine by 30 percent, compared with quieter situations.

Try: Adding more pleasing sounds to your environment with your favorite CDs or a set of wind chimes. It might seem like you're just turning up the volume, but there's a difference between noise (which you consider annoying) and sound (which is pleasing to your ear), says John House, MD, president of the House Ear Institute in Los Angeles.

SEE: GREEN SCENES

A view of nature—whether it's a panoramic vista or a simple houseplant—can lower blood pressure by 11 percent and boost feelings of contentment, studies show.

Try: Opening your shades if you have a garden view; if not, forest and beach pictures have a similar effect. Or scatter potted plants throughout your home.

"Pick plants with rounded leaves. Research suggests gentle, organic shapes may be the most soothing," says Dr. Augustin.

FEEL: AMPLE SPACE

Some experts suggest that humans are hardwired to seek out spaciousness, harking back to our ancestors' need to flee predators. Studies show that mice in cramped conditions exhibit more signs of stress than ones with room to roam.

Try: Taking doors off closed bookcases and filling shelves only halfway, says Arthur Stamps, PhD, president of the Institute of Environmental Quality, a nonprofit research group in San Francisco. Placing a big mirror on one wall is another time-honored trick for making a room seem larger, as is a coat of paint in a cool shade like pale blue, green, or icy white. To mimic airy, outdoor open space, paint ceilings a lighter color than the walls, and position lamps so they throw light on the ceiling.

CHAPTER 24

SEVEN WAYS to Boost Your BRAINPOWER

Prevention *readers who followed this routine boosted everyday memory by up to 78 percent! Try our 4-week game plan today. You won't forget it!*

We've all experienced it: the brain cramp moment. Your mental motor stalls, and you forget the name of the person you just met or struggle to spit out a word hanging on the tip of your tongue. While occasional memory lapses aren't necessarily a cause for concern (they're easily triggered by stress or sleep deprivation), you can take simple steps to prevent them.

Groundbreaking research has revealed specific ways to feel smarter today and keep your mind sharp over time. *Prevention* asked Cynthia R. Green,

PhD, an assistant clinical professor in the department of psychiatry at Mount Sinai School of Medicine and founder of its renowned Memory Enhancement Program, to turn this cutting-edge science into an easy-to-follow guide. The result: the Brainpower Game Plan, a 4-week program that details specific foods and workouts to help you think quickly, clearly, and creatively.

The plan also includes daily brain games. "To keep your brain firing on all cylinders, you need to challenge yourself regularly with mental exercises and new experiences," says Dr. Green. Adults who frequently engage in mentally stimulating activities are 63 percent less likely to develop dementia than those who rarely do such activities, a *New England Journal of Medicine* study discovered. A University of Michigan study found that adults who play a mentally challenging game every day for several weeks can dramatically improve their memory.

The Brainpower Game Plan works. *Prevention* evaluated the cognitive skills of a panel of readers (each received a score called a Brain Q) and put them on the program. After just 4 weeks. scores jumped an average of 28 percent. Some soared even higher—as much as 78 percent.

Start flexing your mental muscles today with our Brainpower program—an inspired regimen you'll want to adopt for life. For more science-backed games, visit www.prevention.com/braingames. (See answers on page 352.)

What's your Brain Q? Get your brainpower score (and see how to boost it) at www.prevention.com/brainfitnessquiz.

BRAIN GAMES WEEK 1

Day 1: Name the style. Challenge your ability to stay focused: Quickly read out loud the style of text used for each word below that the word is printed in—not the word itself. Try it repeatedly to see if you can improve.

Bold	Underlined	**Italic**
Italic	*Regular*	Bold
Underlined	**Italic**	Regular
Regular	Bold	*Underlined*

Day 2: In just 7 words. Test your creativity with this verbal challenge. Write a short story—and use only seven words to tell your tale.

Day 3: Opposite day. Build new neuronal connections by putting your non-dominant hand into action. Use it to perform daily tasks such as brushing your teeth, combing your hair, and eating. Even try to write with your other hand, too. Does using your nondominant hand become any easier over the course of the day?

Day 4: Find it. This teaser will help hone your visual searching skills. The following table features many different symbols. Using 30 seconds for each symbol, count how many times each of the three symbols at the top appears in the table.

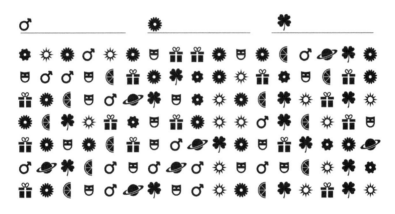

Day 5: Project notes. Get in the habit of taking notes whenever you receive critical information, such as from a doctor or lawyer, or in any circumstance that might cause stress and anxiety, which can cloud your memory. Note taking is always a good idea on the job, too. Try this: Staple several sheets of blank paper to the inside of a project folder and use them to take notes during meetings to produce a clear record of what you discussed.

Day 6: Get the picture. Give your visual attention span a workout. Study the following photograph for 1 minute. Then close the book and write down as many of the items in the photo as you can remember. Try a second time, but before you start, take a deep breath and actively focus on the photo. Did you do any better the second time?

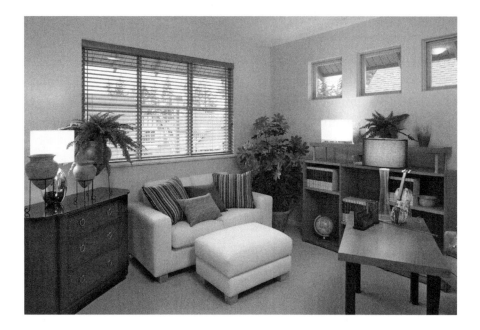

Day 7: Count backward. Here's a brain workout that will help keep your mind on track. Try these three exercises in simple subtraction:

Beginning at 200, count backward, subtracting 5 each time (200, 195, 190 . . .).

Beginning at 150, count backward, subtracting 7 each time (150, 143, 136 . . .).

Beginning at 100, count backward, subtracting 3 each time (100, 97, 94 . . .).

BRAIN GAMES WEEK 2

Day 1. Scent walk. Go for a stroll around your office, your neighborhood, or a local park. Focus on the various scents you encounter along the way.

Day 2. Invent it. Do you have a practical problem that is making you crazy? Spend 10 minutes writing down all the solutions that come to mind. If your idea requires a newly invented gadget, try sketching a few options. This approach is what led to the creation of everything from the potato peeler to the Post-it.

Day 3. Domino effect. Sometimes remembering all the items on a list isn't enough—you need to know them in order, like directions. The domino technique lets the information fall into place. To try it, mentally connect one item on the list with the item that follows it by creating a visual image or phrase in your mind. For instance, if your list was calendar, gloves, shoelaces, and plate, you might start by connecting calendar to gloves by picturing a calendar with photographs of gloves as illustrations. To hook gloves to shoelaces, you might imagine a pair of gloved hands tying a pair of shoes. Now try using the domino technique to remember the following words.

HUT
CANDLE
RECORD
FOOT
POUR
BRUSH
CANDY

Day 4. Master the unspoken word. Learning a foreign language is challenging, particularly as we get older, but using sign language also requires your brain to work in new ways, since you must express yourself using your hands instead of a familiar spoken dialect. Teach yourself the following sign language alphabet, then try to sign some simple sentences to your spouse or friend.

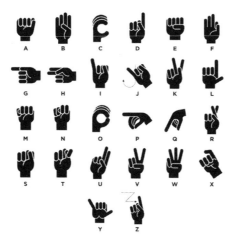

Day 5. Word world. Find as many words as you can in the grid in 3 minutes. Words can run in any direction—up, down, sideways, or diagonally—as long as each letter touches the following letter. For example, you can form the word LARGE by starting with L, moving up to A, diagonally to R, and so on.

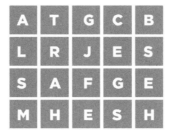

WORK OUT TO STAY SHARP

A workout for your body can also make your brain work better. Here's how. **SHAKE UP YOUR CARDIO.** Just 30 minutes of moderate-intensity exercise 3 times a week can lower your risk of problems such as poor memory and short attention span by up to 20 percent, according to Harvard School of Public Health researchers. For maximum brain boost, inject novelty. Doing different activities throughout the week or even within the same workout (splitting up half an hour into 10 minutes each on a treadmill, elliptical, and bicycle, for example) prevents hitting a mental and physical plateau.

TAKE CHALLENGING CLASSES. Do yoga or dancelike routines, which involve complex movements that require thinking and focus, at least twice a week. A preliminary study found that people who excelled at activities such as these scored exceptionally well on short-term memory tests. Learning new moves stimulates your neurons to grow and create new connections, which results in speedier thinking and sharper memory.

SOCIALIZE WHILE YOU SWEAT. According to a recent study of more than 16,600 adults ages 50 and older, staying connected with others can double memory power. Schedule daily walks with a pal.

Day 6. Sing it. Today, you'll sing for your synapses with a brain stretch that lets you show off your musical side. Create a jingle by putting the following words to music. Don't worry—this isn't a contest. The goal is simple: to challenge your brain (and let you get in the groove).

HEART	SUGAR	PUFF
BOX	RAW	HAIR
MATTER	DANDELION	FOREST

Day 7. Original origami. Take a blank sheet of paper and fold it into an interesting shape. Now start over with a fresh sheet of paper. Try to come up with two or more origami creations. Stumped? Try making a boat or a house.

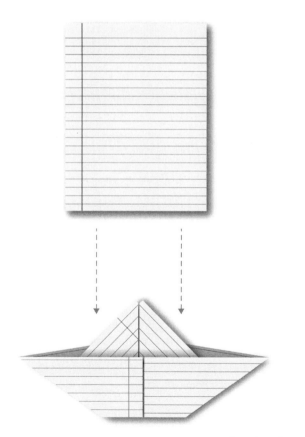

(continued on page 276)

SURPRISING WAYS TO BOOST YOUR BRAIN

Around the time we hit 30, our brains begin a slow, steady downward trajectory—or so popular wisdom would have it. But cognitive decline is by no means an inescapable side effect of aging. In fact, according to a flurry of new reports, you can counteract age-related changes in the brain with a surprisingly simple regimen of activities guaranteed to nurture and fortify your mental muscle power. Here are easy ways to keep your brain quick, sharp, and bristling with youthful vigor.

Google

When you search the Internet, you engage key centers in your brain that control decision making and complex reasoning—and these few clicks may be more mentally stimulating than reading, say UCLA scientists. Their studies found that Internet searching uses neural circuitry that's not activated during reading—but only in people with prior Internet experience. MRI results showed almost 3 times more brain activity in regular Internet searchers than in first-timers, suggesting that repeated Googling can be a great way to build cognitive strength over time.

TIP: Spend around 20 minutes a few days a week searching topics you've always wanted to learn more about—regardless of how seemingly frivolous. Whether you're researching a celebrity's latest pratfalls or musical harmony, the benefits to your brain are the same.

Exercise

Yes, exercise can stave off or delay dementia, but did you know that regular workouts can actually reverse aging in the brain? A team from the University of Illinois' Beckman Institute recently reviewed dozens of past studies and found that aerobic exercise boosts not only speed and sharpness of thought but also the volume of brain tissue.

TIP: As little as 50 minutes of brisk walking 3 times a week was found to have this brain-expanding effect. For an added boost, walk in the park: University of Michigan researchers found that volunteers whose course took them through a tree-filled setting performed 20 percent better on memory and attention tests than those who walked downtown.

Brush and Floss

Here's yet another reason to practice good dental hygiene: Oral health is clearly linked to cognitive health, according to a team of British psychiatrists and dentists. After studying thousands of subjects ages 20 to 59, they found that gingivitis and periodontal disease were associated with worse cognitive function throughout adult life—not just in later years.

TIP: Follow your dentist's advice. Floss daily and brush your teeth for 2 minutes at least once a day.

Drink Sparingly

Keep your alcohol consumption within the safe and healthful limit: no more than one drink a day. The more alcohol a person drinks, the smaller his or her total brain volume becomes, according to a recent Wellesley College study. The link between drinking and reduced brain volume was stronger in women—probably because smaller people are more susceptible to alcohol's effects.

TIP: If you like a glass of white wine with dinner, make a spritzer by replacing some of the wine with sparkling water. You'll cut your intake even more.

Eat Blueberries

New research shows that blueberries may help sharpen your thought processes. After National Institute on Aging and Tufts University researchers injected male rats with kainic acid to simulate the oxidative stress that occurs with aging, rats that had been fed a diet containing 2 percent blueberry extract did better navigating a maze than rats that didn't get the compound. In another study, the same researchers found that rats that ate blueberries showed increased cell growth in the hippocampus region of the brain. The researchers theorize that anthocyanin—the dark blue pigment found in blueberries—is responsible for these cognitive changes. It

(continued)

contains chemicals that may cross the blood-brain barrier and lodge in regions that govern learning and memory.

TIP: Stock up on blueberries when they're on sale, and sprinkle them over your cereal or yogurt or fold them into your smoothie. Off-season, buy them frozen.

Eat Walnuts

USDA researchers have cracked the secret to a younger brain. Simply adding about seven to nine whole nuts to your daily diet may improve balance, coordination, and memory, finds new research in the *British Journal of Nutrition.* Scientists believe the polyphenols and other antioxidants in walnuts help strengthen neural connections and improve cognitive skills.

TIP: Eat a small handful of walnuts each day.

Play Sudoku

In a University of Alabama study of nearly 3,000 older men and women, those who participated in ten 60- to 75-minute sessions of this brain-boosting exercise sharpened their mental abilities so much that their brains performed like those of people more than 10 years younger.

TIP: Start small. Whip out a booklet of basic puzzles when you're riding to work on the train or waiting in a long checkout line. As your skills improve, graduate to more challenging brainteasers.

BRAIN GAMES WEEK 3

Day 1. Memory Places. Today, set up a Memory Place. Find a bowl, dish, or other container large enough to hold your keys, wallet, glasses, cell phone—any important object that you are constantly picking up and putting down. Set up your Memory Place near the front door or whichever entry you use most often. Now cultivate the positive habit of always putting those frequently lost objects in your Memory Place. Here's another useful idea—keep a pad of

Meditate

More than just a great stress reliever, meditation can also enhance your gray matter, says a new study from Massachusetts General Hospital in Boston. Participants appear to have experienced growth in the cortex, which is an area of the brain that controls memory, language, and sensory processing. In addition, meditators in a University of Kentucky study performed better than their nonmeditating counterparts on a series of mental acuity tests.

TIP: Make the practice a regular habit. The participants in a recent study meditated an average of 40 minutes a day. But you can start with 15 on your lunch break or before you leave for work. Sit upright, close your eyes, and focus on whatever you're experiencing in the present moment, whether it's birds chirping in the distance or just the sound of your own breathing.

Drink Coffee

These mental benefits are good to the last drop: Middle-age adults who drink 3 to 5 cups of caffeinated coffee a day are 65 to 70 percent less likely to develop dementia more than 2 decades later, compared with consumers of up to 2 cups, reports a Swedish study. Coffee's magnesium, antioxidants, and caffeine may contribute to its protective effects, say the researchers.

TIP: Just say yes to Starbucks.

sticky notes and a pen in your Memory Place. That way, when you remember something you need to take with you (like the dry cleaning or a DVD to return), you can write yourself a note and stick it on the door.

Day 2. Relate it. With this memory strategy, the idea is to associate or "link" new information you are learning with a familiar concept (for example: "1024" would become "October 24"). Try it on the numbers below, then close the book and note as many numbers from the list as you can recall.

529

25186

4295014

317492706

1528469537

Day 3. Rebus rally. Each of the word combinations below represents a common phrase. Can you figure out all six? To get you started, we'll give you the first one: "Big bad wolf." Can you see why?*

1. BAD wolf

2. S

   L

   O

   W

3. R | E | A | D

4. EGGS

   EASY

5. TOUKEEPCH

6. SCOTCH

   ROCKS

Day 4. Compose a limerick. A limerick is a humorous five-line poem in which the first, second, and fifth lines rhyme with one another and have the same number of syllables (typically, eight or nine). The third and fourth lines rhyme with each other and are shorter in length (typically, five or six syllables). We'll give you the first line: "There once was a gal who was brainy." Can you finish the limerick? You don't have to be Irish to know this is more than just fun. It's zany!

Day 5. Word maker. Using one set of information in different ways tests your brain's flexibility. How many words can you make out of each of the following words?

BALDERDASH

CACOPHONY

ONOMATOPOEIA

Day 6. Sound walk. Continue to explore the role your senses play in how your brain perceives the world. Go for a stroll around your office, your neighborhood, or a local park. Notice the various sounds you hear along the way.

Day 7. Picture/Repicture it. Hone your brain's visual flexibility by learning to look at the same object from different perspectives. Can you picture this? And that? Each of these three pictures depicts two very different images, depending on how you look at it. Can you see both?

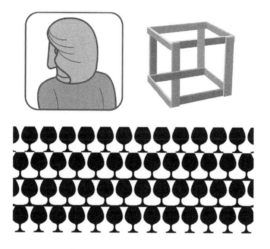

BRAIN GAMES WEEK 4

Day 1. Triangles. See how many triangles you can find in the picture below.

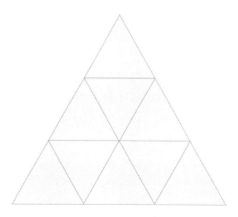

Day 2. Hello, friend. Call a friend you haven't spoken with in at least 3 years. As you reminisce, you'll probably end up talking about mutual friends you knew in the old days, which is a great booster for your memory bank.

Day 3. Color with crayons. Recapture the joy of pure creativity. When was the last time you had some fun with crayons—with or without a coloring book? Get a few sheets of blank paper and start coloring. You might be surprised by what you come up with.

Day 4. Concentration. Lay out a deck of playing cards facedown on a table. Turning over two cards at a time, try to find matching pairs. If the two you turn over don't match, return them to the table facedown. If you make a match, remove the cards. Obviously, at first you won't make many pairs, but trying to remember where cards are located will help you clear the table. (If you want to start out by making the game easier, use only half the deck, leaving one pair of each number and face card.) Use a stopwatch and see how long it takes to find all the pairs.

Day 5. Name it. Using scrap paper, write down as many types of animals as you can think of in 1 minute. How did you do? Did you remember albatross and zebra? Now try this exercise again, only this time with types of fruit. When you're done, try the exercise one more time, choosing your own category—car models, perhaps, or dog breeds.

Day 6. Junk drawer jam. Take inventory of your junk drawer for a visual memory workout. Open the drawer and study the cluttered contents for 1 minute. Then close the drawer and write down as many of the items inside as you can recall. Want a brain-boosting bonus? Reorganize the drawer, tossing out stuff that's truly junk.

Day 7. Decode this. Using the following cipher, decode the message below.

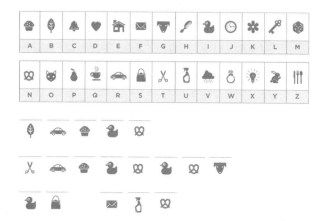

CHAPTER 25

ENERGY FOR LIFE

Increase your energy levels and shrink your belly in minutes a day with a totally new way of moving.

What if you could boost your energy levels—not to mention flatten your belly, strengthen your back, and improve your flexibility—in just minutes a day, without even standing up? That's the genius behind Gyrokinesis, which is a seated workout that combines the core-strengthening benefits of Pilates, the flexibility of yoga, the grace of dance, the fluidity of swimming, and the energy lift of tai chi in one simple, dynamic routine.

"Most types of exercise use linear motions—forward and back or side to side. Gyrokinesis is more about three-dimensional movements, including spirals and circles," explains Justine Bernard, DPT, a physical therapist in Washington, DC. These actions better mimic the way your body moves in everyday life to target more muscles—including your deepest abs—and work your joints in a greater range of motion.

Gyrokinesis was created in the late '70s by Juliu Horvath, a former ballet dancer from Romania, after he suffered a career-ending injury. While it's helped many dancers, including Bernard, recover from debilitating injuries, the practice is growing and helping even nondancers. Ten years ago, there were only about 175 studios worldwide offering Gyrokinesis; today, there are more than 2,000, and 6,200 instructors.

Unlike yoga, which requires a certain amount of strength and flexibility, Gyrokinesis can be done while sitting on a low stool or chair, making it easy for people at any fitness level and a perfect at-your-desk workout. And doing flowing movements increases your heart rate and breathing to carry more energizing oxygen throughout your body.

"When I did it in the morning, it gave me a big boost that stayed with me for hours," says Avery Brandon, 41, of New York City, one of our readers who road-tested our 15-minute routine for 2 weeks.

This workout was designed by Justine Bernard, DPT, physical therapist, Gyrokinesis master trainer, and owner of Elements Fitness and Wellness Center in Washington, DC.

PREVENTION Alert!

SHORTCUT TO MEGA ENERGY

Good news for your craziest days: As little as 10 minutes of daily walking (or 25 minutes just 3 days a week) boosted exercisers' energy scores by about 18 percent, according to a study by the Pennington Biomedical Research Center.

Do you have more time? Keep going for an even bigger energy blast. If you walk for 20 minutes, you'll get a blast of pep that lasts all day, reveals new research from the University of Vermont. Though exercise provides an immediate lift, scientists were surprised at the long-lasting effect, because mood-boosting endorphins stay elevated for only a couple of hours. Researchers speculate that the jump-start helps buffer the effects of everyday hassles and stress on your outlook throughout the day.

EAT SMART FOR ALL-DAY ENERGY

To put pep in your step and stay mentally sharp, eat less fat. A British study found that rats fed a diet of 55 percent total fat experienced a 50 percent drop in exercise stamina and significant short-term memory loss in as little as 9 days, compared with rats fed a low-fat diet. A "high-fat hangover" reduces heart and muscle efficiency, say researchers. Eat for maximum energy: Keep total fat intake between 20 and 35 percent of your daily calories—about 35 to 62 grams of fat—with most coming from the monounsaturated fatty acids in fish, nuts, and seeds.

Our seated Gyrokinesis workout includes 3 series of exercises. You can do them all together for a total-body energizer or spread them throughout the day for on-the-spot pick-me-ups. Along with avoiding the afternoon slump, you'll stand taller, feel tighter, and notice fewer aches and pains—in just 2 weeks.

WORKOUT AT A GLANCE

What you'll need: A stool or armless chair

What to do: Complete each series (Abs and Back, page 288; Legs and Hips, page 290; and Upper Body, page 291) three times, then move on to the next. Keep the motion smooth, breathing deeply through your nose.

How often: Do the workout 3 to 7 days a week. It's a perfect get-started routine for beginners. If you already exercise, you can use it as a warm-up.

SERIES 1: ABS AND BACK

Tones your core and increases spinal flexibility. Do each exercise 4 times (on each side when appropriate), moving smoothly from start to finish, before going on to the next. Repeat the series 3 times.

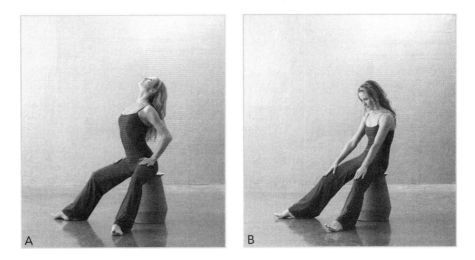

⌃ ARCH AND CURL

Sit with feet more than hip-width apart, toes out, hands on thighs. Inhale and arch spine, lifting chest and gazing at ceiling (A). Keep shoulders over hips. Exhale. Inhale and sit up, lengthening spine. Keep abs pulled in throughout. Exhale and round spine forward, looking at floor about 6 feet in front of you, feeling a stretch in low back (B). Don't let chin drop to chest. Inhale as you sit up.

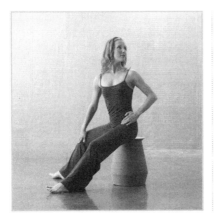

⟨ SPIRAL

Sit tall, hands on thighs. Inhale as you lengthen spine, pulling in abdominals. Exhale and rotate torso to left as far as comfortable, sliding left hand to hip, eyes gazing over left shoulder. Inhale as you return to center. Repeat, switching hands as you rotate to right.

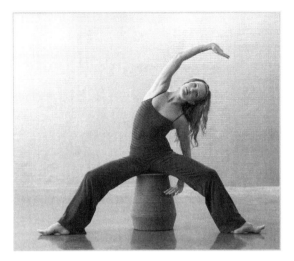

⌃ SIDE ARCH

Sit tall with legs wide. Inhale as you lengthen spine and pull in abdominals. Exhale and reach right arm out to side, then overhead, bending to left (left hand presses toward floor). Push left foot into floor, feeling stretch along right side. Inhale as you hold. Exhale and return to center; inhale. Repeat with left arm, bending to right and pressing right foot into floor.

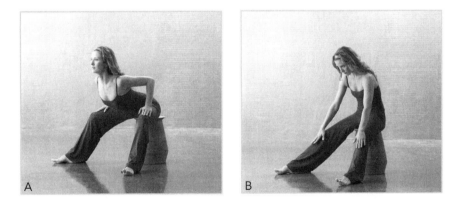

⌃ WAVE

Sit tall with hands on thighs, feet wide. Inhale, arching spine; exhale lower torso toward floor as far as you comfortably can, keeping back arched (A). Round spine, curling up one vertebra at a time (B), as you inhale and lengthen spine, returning to start position.

SERIES 2: LEGS AND HIPS

Strengthens your abs and legs and stretches your hips to prevent or reduce knee and back pain. Do all 3 moves first with the left leg, then with the right, 1 time each. Repeat, completing the series 3 times.

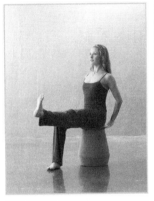

⊙ LEG EXTENSION

Sit tall on edge of stool, feet flat on floor, hands on seat back for support, fingers pointing forward. Inhale, then exhale and extend left leg, foot flexed, knee toward ceiling, heel reaching forward. Hold and inhale. Keep abdominals tight throughout.

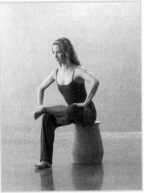

⊙ CROSS OVER

From Leg Extension, exhale and cross left ankle over right knee, keeping foot flexed; place hands on bent leg for support. With abs tight, lean forward, gently pressing on left thigh.

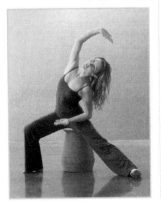

⊙ SIDE KICK

From Cross Over, inhale back into Leg Extension with left leg, foot flexed. Exhale, bend leg back in, and extend to left side like you're kicking. Lower flexed foot so inside edge is on floor, knee pointing forward. Place left arm on left thigh, palm up. Reach right arm overhead, palm up, and bend to left, feeling a stretch on right side of torso and left inner thigh. Hold for a second, then return to starting position. Repeat series from beginning, this time with right leg.

SERIES 3: UPPER BODY

Stretches upper back and shoulders to improve posture. Do each move 4 times, as described, and complete the series 3 times.

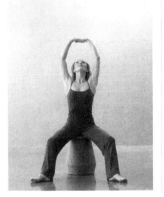

⊙ OVERHEAD CIRCLES

Sit tall with legs wide, toes pointing out. Interlace fingers, reaching arms overhead as you inhale, palms facing ceiling, elbows slightly bent, abs tight. Exhale as you bend to right side, keeping arms overhead, and circle forward, rounding spine. Inhale as you circle to left and back, arching spine. Circle 4 times, moving in a fluid motion with abs tight. Repeat, circling in the opposite direction 4 times.

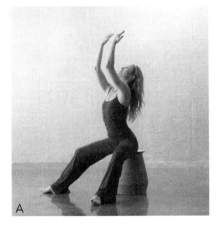

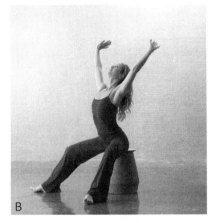

⊙ BIG YAWNS

Sit tall, hands on thighs, legs wide. Inhale and reach arms forward and up overhead, palms facing body; gently arch spine (A). Straighten and rotate arms so palms face forward and arms are open wide, reaching toward sky (B). Exhale and circle arms back and down. Do 4 times.

CHAPTER 26

THE FAMILY
Sleep Cure

Everyone tosses and turns for different reasons. Here's how to make sure the whole clan gets the z's they need to stay happy and healthy.

Your husband is on his third cup of coffee, and it's not yet 8 a.m. Your teen is so bleary-eyed and grumpy that you want to run in the other direction. And you are so tired you can barely remember your middle name.

If your family is like most, everyone is seriously sleep deprived. A study from the CDC found that only 1 out of 3 Americans gets enough sleep all month long. And 16 percent of adults get less than 6 hours per night, says the National Sleep Foundation. That's well short of the 7 to 8 hours needed to ward off obesity, high blood pressure, and other ills. To complicate matters, each family member deals with unique sleep sappers, says Susan Zafarlotfi, PhD, clinical director of the Institute for Sleep-Wake Disorders at Hackensack University Medical Center. But these simple strategies will help your family sleep longer and better every night.

DREAM UP BETTER HEALTH

If you're like most people, your return to consciousness each morning follows a predictable pattern: You blink awake, still half-trapped in the dream you just had—a high-stakes epic in which you soared over the Grand Canyon or watched as a tsunami engulfed your house. What was *that* about? Within minutes, though, you sweep away the hallucinatory traces like cobwebs, dismissing the dream as just another meaningless, though exciting, sleep-time drama.

But hold on: New science suggests you're passing up a great opportunity to gain a little self-knowledge. Experts say our brains' nocturnal sagas can supply us with insights that will help heal emotional stress and trauma, enable us to sleep better, make us feel happier while awake, or even answer nagging questions about our lives. How? Thoughts that occur while you sleep mingle recent events, buried memories, and hopes and fears into a potent stew, forging neural connections that might never be made through conscious thought alone.

"The latest brain research suggests that dreams are part of a healthy emotional coping process," says dream researcher Robert Hoss, author of *Dream Language*.

Indeed, recent brain-scan studies show that regions active during dreaming are the same ones responsible for processing memories and emotions when we're awake. Dreams, the new thinking goes, shape your self-image by helping you work through unresolved emotions from waking life. (For this reason, even unpleasant nightmares can be beneficial, says Hoss.) In fact, for a day or two after a significant life event—and again about a week later—hints of it show up in your dreams, according to a study at Canada's University of Alberta.

"Revisiting events in dreams helps reshape your understanding of them," says study author Don Kuiken, PhD.

With a little know-how, you can reap these insights on your own. Here are three strategies that will help you benefit from your subconscious mind's nocturnal adventures.

WAKE UP SLOWLY. Your conscious mind can wipe away memories of a dream in minutes—and with them, possible insights. To prevent images from slipping away too quickly, lie still in bed right after waking up, keeping your eyes closed and concentrating on what you were just dreaming about, suggests Charles McPhee, former director of the sleep apnea treatment program at the Sleep Disorders Center of Santa Barbara, California, and author of *Ask the Dream Doctor.* When you've recalled everything you can, jot down the dream's details in a notebook kept by your bed. Come back to this entry later to think more about what your dream might have been telling you, and look for recurring characters, places, and patterns over time.

DON'T TAKE IT LITERALLY. Straightforward dream interpretations seldom yield insight. If you subconsciously imagine kissing your friend's brother, for example, it doesn't necessarily mean you want to betray your spouse. Tufts University professor of psychiatry Ernest Hartmann, MD, confirmed this idea when he studied Americans' dreams after the terrorist attacks of September 11, 2001. "The dreams had more intense, powerful images"—like frightening animals, for instance—"than ones before 9/11, but almost none were about the Twin Towers themselves," he says. Rather than take dreams at face value, try a little free association to get at their real meaning. For example, what's your first impression of your friend's brother? If "gregarious" comes to mind, you could be longing for a more active social life.

CONFRONT YOUR "DEMONS." People who experience trauma in their lives often relive it while asleep, but eventually they acquire "mastery" in their dreams, meaning they find a way to take charge of unpleasant subconscious images. Patrick Andries, a dream therapist and cofounder of the School of Intuitive Arts and Sciences in Illinois, recalls one client who had a recurring nightmare that she was being chased by a mysterious woman. "She finally decided to stand up to this person," Andries recalls. "When she asked her in the dream, 'Who are you?' the dream character replied, 'I'm your low self-esteem.'" This insight enabled Andries's client to move forward and better appreciate her unique abilities. To develop a similar take-charge mind-set, try "dream intervention." If you take control of your dreams, your dream content may soon become less stressful, says Andries.

QUICK! RUN TO BED!

One of the many benefits of exercise is cancer prevention, but getting too little shut-eye may cancel out its protective effect, concludes a new study. Researchers tracked nearly 6,000 women for about a decade and found that workout buffs who slept 7 or fewer hours per night had a 50 percent greater chance of developing cancer than exercisers who got more z's—similar to the risk of nonexercisers. Insufficient sleep may cause hormonal and metabolic disturbances linked to cancer risk, erasing the benefits of exercise.

YOUR KIDS

Sleep thief: Late-night gadget time. Artificial light from computer and television screens tells the brain that it's not time to wind down.

"Your body thinks artificial light is daylight, which prevents the release of melatonin, a sleep-inducing chemical," says Dr. Zafarlotfi. A study from Wayne State University found that talking on a cell phone before snoozing caused a 13 percent drop in deep sleep, which is the type that helps people recover from daily wear and tear. Here's how to get your kids to log off.

Set a technology curfew. Shut off the TV and have your children stop using phones and computers at least an hour before bed, advises Dr. Zafarlotfi.

Use the dimmer switch. Turn down the lights in your kids' rooms a half hour before bedtime to allow melatonin to kick in, she says. Or try switching the bulbs in their rooms to 60 watts or less.

Do morning prep at night. Teens, whose biological clocks tend to be on a later sleep cycle, often struggle with early start times at school. Encourage your kids to shower and get clothes and homework ready in the evening, and choose fast breakfasts (such as cereal) so they can sleep in as much as possible.

MOM

Sleep thief: Stress. Anxiety and other frazzled states cause a woman's body to release adrenaline, a brain chemical that triggers alertness, says sleep specialist Joyce Walsleben, PhD, associate professor of medicine at New York University.

Adds Dr. Zafarlotfi: "Stress seems to keep more women awake than men, which explains why 90 percent of my patients are female." Here's how to ease your mind.

Shower an hour before bed. The warm water is relaxing. Plus, your body temperature will dip afterward, mimicking the physiological changes that naturally occur before sleep.

Write away worries. During the day, scribble down your concerns and how you plan to handle them, advises Dr. Walsleben. For example, if you're

---

YOUR COMMON DREAMS DECIPHERED

Although every dream (and dreamer) is unique, many themes crop up repeatedly. Here are three dreams many people have, and possible interpretations from experts.

FLYING. This is usually a good dream—a sign that you're in control of your life. The more skillfully you maneuver through the air, the more likely you are to feel in charge of things while awake. On the other hand, if your airborne self gets buffeted by winds, the dream could suggest a loss of control.

TEETH FALLING OUT. Because teeth "process" food just as the brain digests new knowledge, losing your teeth can mean you've come across information that you aren't quite ready to accept yet, dream therapist Patrick Andries says.

FAILING A SCHOOL TEST. This dream typically occurs when you are feeling tested by a life circumstance. Ask yourself how you are being challenged or judged, and what you can do to relax and effectively prepare for what (or whom) you're facing.

PREVENTION
Alert!

THE POWER SLEEP HOUR

Sleeping 8 hours per night (instead of 7 or less) can make you about 30 percent less likely to develop a cold, according to Carnegie Mellon University researchers. Participants who reported difficulty falling asleep or not feeling rested the next morning also had decreased immunity.

panicked about bills, you might write that you'll go through them and come up with a payment schedule for those you can't tackle right away. Then, if you start to ruminate before lights-out, tell yourself firmly, "I've already dealt with this. It's time to go to sleep."

Make exercise a habit. Getting your heart rate up for 20 minutes every day—by walking, gardening, or cleaning the house—can lower anxiety and stress levels by as much as 40 percent, according to a study of about 20,000 adults at University College in London.

DAD

Sleep thief: Snoring. By age 50, half of men snore, says Michael Thorpy, MD, director of the Sleep-Wake Disorders Center at Montefiore Medical Center in New York City.

"The noise can actually wake him up," he says, or prevent him from getting into deeper, more restorative sleep stages. Here's how to stop the noise.

Measure your neck. "A big neck increases the odds that breathing during sleep will be interrupted," says Charles Bae, MD, a neurologist and sleep specialist with the Cleveland Clinic in Ohio. One reason: If a man's neck is bigger than 17 inches, it might indicate excess weight, which puts pressure on the airways and can lead to snoring.

Skip wine with dinner. If you like to wind down with a drink, make sure your last cocktail is at least 3 hours before bed. Alcohol relaxes the throat, which makes snoring worse, says Dr. Thorpy.

Get help. If you have tried everything and still feel exhausted during the day or are falling asleep during work (or while driving!), get checked for sleep apnea, a condition in which breathing is blocked for seconds at a time. The disorder prevents the body from getting enough oxygen during sleep and raises the risk of heart attacks and strokes. You're also more likely to have high blood pressure and erectile dysfunction if you have sleep apnea.

Don't go sleep on the couch. A man is more likely to stick with sleep treatment if his wife shares his bed, finds a study from Rush University. Earplugs or a white-noise machine can muffle the din of severe snoring. Try to nod off together.

THE GRANDPARENTS

Sleep thief: Changing circadian rhythms. As people get older, hormonal and brain changes cause a shift in the body's internal clock, so they might find themselves sleepy very early in the evening.

"This starts a vicious cycle," says Dr. Zafarlotfi. "If they go to bed at 8, they may rise at 3 or 4 in the morning. Then they take long naps. So when bedtime rolls around, they're not tired enough to doze off, which deprives them of deep sleep." To help seniors snooze on schedule, suggest that they:

Skip catnaps. They should try to get all 8 hours of sleep at one time—or, if they must take a nap, have them set an alarm so they sleep no more than 20 to 30 minutes.

PREVENTION
→ **Alert!**

VENT BEFORE YOU HIT THE HAY

For better-quality shut-eye, express your anger before you head to bed. Researchers found that heart patients who stifle angry feelings are twice as likely to report poor sleep quality as those who share them. Both too little sleep and roiling emotions can elevate stress hormones, taking a toll on overall health. "Many people are afraid to express anger to their partner or friends," says study author Mary Whooley, MD. "Start by stating how you feel instead of attacking or criticizing."

THE SECRET TO WAKING UP HAPPY

Go to bed—and get up—early. New Brazilian research found that night owls are nearly 3 times more likely to experience depression symptoms than early birds, even when they get the same amount of sleep. Experts aren't sure exactly why, but there may be an optimal time within the 24-hour clock to fall asleep and wake up, says sleep expert Lisa Shives, MD. "Going to bed late can be bad for your mood and your overall health."

Stick to light fare. Recent animal studies suggest that a high-fat diet can disrupt circadian rhythms. Though further research is needed, "greasy, heavy dinners and desserts may disrupt digestion, so you toss and turn," says Dr. Bae.

Turn up the light. Unlike teens, seniors may benefit from bright light exposure in the evening. It keeps them from falling asleep too early, explains Dr. Bae. Look for full-spectrum bulbs, which mimic natural daylight.

"MY FATHER'S MUSICAL LIFELINE"

I can hear my father whistling as I write this.

by Mary Ellen Geist

Because of Alzheimer's disease, my father doesn't know what day it is. He doesn't know my name. But when he sings, I have my dad back again.

The aide who answered the phone in the Alzheimer's unit shouted, "Woody, you've got a phone call!" I heard the clattering as he grasped the handset, followed by his whistle, a nervous habit he acquired over the past few years. "It's Mary Ellen, your daughter," I said. Then I hummed him a note, as if I were giving him a cue from the pitch pipe—and began to sing "Moon River." By the second note, he was right on beat. My father can't remember the names of people he once knew, what year it is, or how old he is, but he can still recall all the lyrics to this and almost every song he has ever sung. We sang "Moon River" through to the end.

When I left my career as a broadcast journalist nearly 4 years ago to help my mother care for him, I was shocked by his condition. Some mornings, he was a shell of a person. But when there was music, he responded. So I devised my own therapy regimen: We stood in front of a mirror and sang one of the songs he had performed for more than 4 decades with an a cappella group called the Grunyons. With some urging, he watched himself sing—and something remarkable happened: He stood up straighter, looking into the mirror as if we were on stage. His face changed as he became more lucid and seemed to recall the man he once was—the man who loved to perform; the man who ran a distribution company, who gave speeches, who took control.

My mother and I used special songs during the day: We woke him with Frank Sinatra's version of "In the Wee Small Hours of the Morning." I'd start the CD, and he'd hum while his eyes were still closed. More rousing tunes cheered him up during the day, and at night, we'd go with softer hymns like "Now the Day Is Over." When there was no music, he'd whistle. It was how he created his own soundtrack.

In January 2008, after much discussion, we put Dad in a nearby assisted living residence. Even though I shared in the caregiving duties, Mom had done it alone for more than a decade, and my sisters and I worried about her. My father needed constant attention; she was nearing 80 years old and was drained, emotionally and physically.

The night we brought him, a party was under way—musical notes hung from the ceiling, and a jazz band played. My father twirled my mother and several residents around the floor. After, he said he was tired, so we told him, "You can go to bed here!" Though we were devastated, he seemed comfortable. So we accompanied him to his room and put on a CD. He was snoring in no time.

We stayed for several days, helping him adjust. Finally, we took an entire day off—the first in the 14 years since my father was diagnosed. When we returned, we found him sitting in a corner, arms crossed over his chest, whistling loudly. The residents were steering a wide path around him; one man yelled, "Don't let him near me, or I'll stuff a rag in his mouth!"

We had forgotten about the whistling. My mother clocked him once: 10 hours straight. We had become so inured to the sound that we didn't think to warn the residents. It annoyed his neighbors and caused feedback in some of their hearing aids.

Within 2 weeks, the management decided to move my father to a floor with residents in the late stages of Alzheimer's disease—many of whom were catatonic. At first, I visited almost every day. I'd play CDs or call to sing with him—music was the only thing that made him smile. But as time passed, the smiles dwindled. My father stopped initiating conversations, lost weight, and wouldn't walk.

Later, I took a freelance job further away, so I could only see him every other week. One day I called to say I was coming to visit. "How are you?" I asked. Without a pause he said, "I'm dead."

It sent shivers through me, but I said, "Dad, I'm coming to see you on Father's Day!"

"Don't bother, because I'll be dead," he said.

I started singing one of his favorite songs, but this time, he didn't chime in. There was only silence. In all the ways I've lost my father to Alzheimer's disease, this was the worst—the one place untouched by the disease was now fading. I called my family, and we agreed: He needed to come home.

During his first few weeks of living with us again, we had to be vigilant—playing CDs or singing constantly; otherwise he might retreat. Even now, more than 6 months later, he gets extremely agitated when someone talks over the music.

One weekend, we took my father to see the University of Michigan's glee club perform. He used to sing with the club, so they invited him to sing "In College Days" with them. Though the words didn't come as easily as they once had, he eventually looked out at the audience, and I saw that only-when-he's-singing smile.

Each night, my mother puts my father to bed in the room they share below the office where I write. He bursts into song, even after he's deep in sleep. Two weeks ago, he sang "Lazy River" over and over the entire night.

I am so glad he's home with us now.

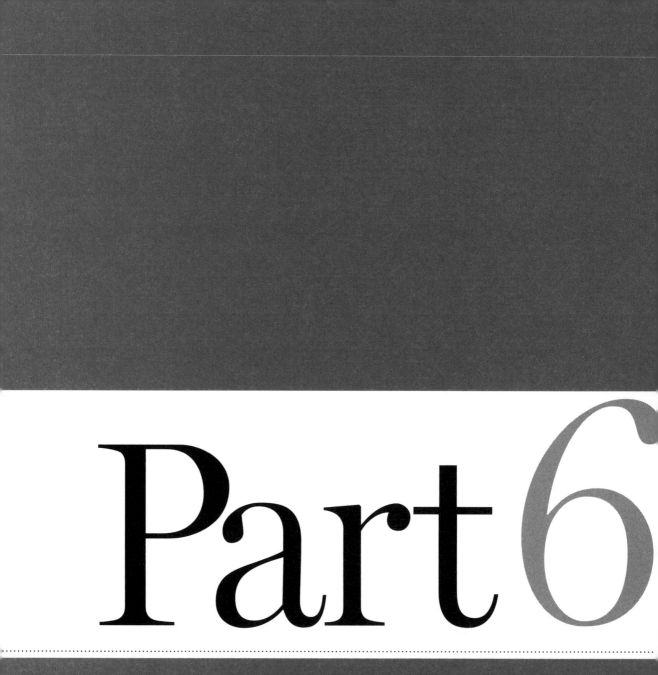

Part 6

BEAUTY
BASICS

CHAPTER 27

Countdown to GREAT SKIN

Look better and brighter in a day, week, or month. Our pro tips will work with any schedule.

Time was, when you needed an instant beauty boost, you slapped on a clay mask and a few cucumber slices and hoped for the best. Thankfully, times have changed. Whether you have a special event on the horizon or need to look spectacular for an important work presentation overnight, there are dozens of high- and low-tech solutions that can smooth wrinkles, reduce redness, and impart a healthy glow. Here's what experts say you can truly accomplish in 1 day, 1 week, and 1 month. Find the timeline that works for your schedule, then choose your main goal; follow the recommended routine, and you'll be wowed by the results!

YOU'VE GOT 1 DAY

You want to look brighter. The night before, use an at-home peel or microdermabrasion kit.

"These products whisk away dead cells and instantly reveal healthier skin," says Elizabeth Briden, MD, adjunct associate clinical professor of dermatology at the University of Minnesota. Bonus: Cosmetics glide on smoother and more evenly.

Try: Avon Anew Clinical Advanced Retexturizing Peel ($25, avon.com) and Neutrogena Healthy Skin Rejuvenator ($40, drugstores).

You want to soften wrinkles. One hour before your event, exfoliate and add moisture; the combination offers immediate plumping that lasts several hours.

"Even gentle sloughing causes skin to swell slightly, making wrinkles less noticeable," says Dr. Briden. Use a scrub with smooth, spherical beads that polish without causing redness (look for polyethylene at the top of the ingredient list). Follow with a lotion that contains GABA, a peptide that relaxes muscles and temporarily eases pesky lines.

Try: 24.7 Skincare Smoothing Anti-Aging Moisturizer ($20, CVS) or DermaFreeze365 ($30, Rite Aid).

You want to lessen redness. In the morning, wash with a mild, soap-free cleanser; pat dry to avoid inflaming skin. Spot treat ruddy areas with a soothing 1 percent over-the-counter hydrocortisone cream or a calming cream.

Throughout the day, skip flare-up items like hot beverages, alcohol, and anything spicy. They release a chemical called histamine that can turn skin red. One hour before your event, apply a washcloth soaked in cold water to your face for 10 minutes; the cool compress constricts blood vessels. Follow with a lotion that boasts a greenish tint.

5 THE AVERAGE TIME, IN MINUTES, IT TAKES NAILS TO DRY UNDER A FAN, ACCORDING TO OPI PRODUCTS

"Green cancels out redness because it's on the opposite end of the color spectrum," says Dr. Briden.

Try: Clinique Redness Solutions Daily Protective Base SPF 15 ($17.50; clinique.com) or Murad Redness Therapy Correcting Moisturizer SPF 15 ($37; murad.com).

YOU'VE GOT 1 WEEK

You want to fade brown spots. At the start of the week, if it's in your budget, try a single session with a Q-Switched Laser, which zaps away unwanted clusters of brown pigment; a scab forms and spots fall off within a few days. Cost: about $250.

Nightly, use a peel or microdermabrasion kit to slough off the top layer of skin, making brown spots less noticeable. Any subsequent redness should be gone by morning.

You want to soften deep lines. Seven days before, get Botox (around $500) to prevent muscle movement that causes crow's feet and forehead furrows; the smoothing effect kicks in within a few days and lasts up to 4 months.

At the same time, instantly plump deep lines and folds with filling materials like Restylane or Juvéderm. Made with hyaluronic acid, a substance found

(continued on page 312)

ARE YOU YOUR SKIN'S FRIEND OR FOE?

You may feel 40 and fabulous (and you are!), but your skin may actually be older. Lifestyle habits can make or break the actual age of your skin, for better or worse. How you care for your complexion is key, too. Grab a pencil and take our quiz. Then use our science-proven tips to stop—and reverse—premature aging.

1. How often do you wash your face?

    a) Just in the evening

    b) Every morning and night

    c) Erratically—sometimes not at all

2. What best describes your sun-protection habits?

    a) I wear sunscreen or a moisturizer with built-in SPF 30 on all exposed areas

    b) I think there's an SPF 15 already in my day cream

    c) I save sunscreen for summertime trips to the beach so I don't burn

3. How well do you handle stress?

    a) My friends say I'm a rock

    b) Okay. I feel frazzled on busy days, but otherwise I'm on an even keel

    c) Not well. It seems I'm always worrying about something

4. True or false: You use a retinoid.

    a) True

    b) False

5. When was the last time you changed your skin care routine?

    a) About 6 months ago

    b) So long ago, I can't remember

    c) Routine? Who has time for that?

6. True or false: Your diet is rich in healthy unsaturated fats.

    a) True

    b) False

7. You exercise:

   a) Regularly—at least 3 times a week

   b) Infrequently—whenever I can squeeze in a workout

   c) Never

Your Score

For every "a" and "true" answer, give yourself 2 points. Each "b" is worth 1 point, and each "c" and "false" is worth zero points.

10 to 14 points: Great job! You're very skin savvy. But keep reading this section anyway to ensure your skin looks as healthy as possible.

5 to 9 points: Not bad, but follow our tips starting on page 312. If you make the appropriate tweaks to your routine and lifestyle, your skin will look brighter, smoother, and firmer in about a month.

0 to 4 points: Uh-oh. You're not doing your skin any favors! Luckily, it is never too late to break bad habits and begin to rejuvenate skin. Use the info in this section to learn how.

YOUR YOUNGER-SKIN STRATEGY

Here are the top seven ways to fight aging—every step of the way.

WASH AT NIGHT. "The most important time to clean your face is before you hit the sack," says Doris Day, MD, New York City-based dermatologist and assistant clinical professor of dermatology at New York University Langone Medical Center.

Dirt, bacteria, and makeup left on overnight can irritate skin, clog pores, and trigger breakouts. Remove this top layer of grime with a gentle face wash (skin should feel pleasantly tight for 10 to 15 minutes post-cleansing), which also allows anti-agers to penetrate deeper for better results. Because oil production dips with hormonal changes in your 40s, cleansing twice daily can dry out your complexion and make wrinkles look more pronounced. To refresh skin in the morning, splash with lukewarm water.

BE VIGILANT ABOUT UV PROTECTION. Nothing is more important than wearing sunscreen (ideally, SPF 30) if you want younger-looking skin. Even 10 minutes of daily exposure to UVA "aging" rays can cause changes that lead to wrinkles and sun spots in as few as 12 weeks. If your moisturizer isn't formulated with a built-in broad-spectrum SPF 30 sunscreen, be sure to apply one daily to block both UVA and UVB rays.

MANAGE STRESS. Emotional upheavals can make your skin look 5 years older than your chronological age, says New York City dermatologist and psychiatrist Amy Wechsler, MD, author of *The Mind-Beauty Connection.* Constant anxiety increases the stress hormone cortisol, which causes inflammation that breaks down collagen. It also triggers a chain of responses that can lead to facial redness and acne flare-ups. To quell inflammation, eat antioxidant-rich foods such as berries, oranges, and asparagus. When you're feeling tense, Dr. Wechsler recommends a few minutes of deep breathing (inhale through your nose, hold for 3 counts, and release through your mouth).

USE A RETINOID. Research shows that these vitamin-A derivatives speed cell turnover and collagen growth to smooth fine lines and wrinkles and fade brown spots. Prescription-strength retinoids such as Renova provide the fastest results. You'll start to see changes in about a month. To help skin acclimate to any redness and peeling, apply just a pea-size drop to your face every third night, building up to nightly usage. Milder OTC versions (look for retinol) are gentler, although it can take up to 3 months to see noticeable results.

UPDATE YOUR SKIN CARE ROUTINE. Changing even one thing in your regimen every 6 to 12 months jump-starts more impressive improvements in tone and texture. "When you apply products consistently, your skin slides into maintenance mode after about a year," says Mary P. Lupo, MD, New Orleans dermatologist and clinical professor of dermatology at Tulane University School of Medicine. To keep it primed for rejuvenation, substitute a cream that contains alpha hydroxy acids for your prescription retinoid twice a week to boost the benefits. Or bump up your OTC retinoid to an Rx formula.

EAT OMEGA-3s. These "good fats" in foods such as salmon, flaxseed, and almonds boost hydration, which keeps skin supple and firm. The same isn't true of the saturated fat in dairy products and meats, which increase free-radical damage that makes skin more susceptible to aging. Limit saturated fat intake to about 17 grams daily.

EXERCISE REGULARLY. Studies find that women who work out regularly have firmer skin than similar non-exercisers. The reason: Exercise infuses skin with oxygen and nutrients needed for collagen production. To keep your skin toned, make time for at least three 30-minute heart-pumping workouts per week.

in skin, these options offer natural-looking fullness for about 6 months. Or try Evolence, which is a new product derived from pig collagen. Due to its thicker consistency, results might last up to a year. Such fast results come at a price: Expect to pay about $600 per treated area. Be prepared for mild swelling and bruising that last a few days.

You want to clear broken capillaries. Seven days before, try the Pulsed Dye Laser, which emits a beam of light that targets red pigment in the skin, causing vessels to collapse. You might experience slight swelling that lingers for 24 to 48 hours. Treatment starts at $150.

Nightly, use a topical retinoid to strengthen weak vein walls. Wait 2 days if you've had the laser.

Daily, apply an SPF of at least 15 (30 is even better) to maintain clearing and prevent the UV damage that often causes the problem in the first place.

YOU'VE GOT 1 MONTH

You want to soften wrinkles and firm skin. Nightly, use a prescription-strength retinoid to target wrinkles all over.

"These vitamin A derivatives supercharge cell turnover, so you'll notice fewer wrinkles by the end of the month," says Arielle Kauvar, MD, a clinical associate professor of dermatology at New York University Langone Medical Center.

Ask your doctor for Atralin, the most moisturizing retinoid, which you can use daily for faster results with minimal dryness or flaking. Caveat: If your skin is sensitive or prone to redness, you might be able to tolerate using the cream only every second or third night, at least for the first 2 weeks.

Every morning, apply a broad-spectrum SPF 30 to protect fresh cells.

You want to look brighter and erase brown spots. Every other week, alternate between using an at-home peel and a microdermabrasion product to fade splotches, reduce fine lines, and boost radiance.

"Combining exfoliators is like power washing your complexion," says Dr. Briden. Follow directions on the label so that you don't strip away too much of your skin's protective outer layer. You might experience some immediate redness, which should dissipate the next day.

Every morning, use a broad-spectrum SPF 30 sunscreen to keep fresh cells from repigmenting.

Nightly, apply a prescription-strength hydroquinone bleaching cream; top with a prescription retinoid to drive the lightener into the skin for faster results. Limit use to 2 months.

Two weeks before, if you can afford to splurge, an in-office peel employing a low level of trichloroacetic acid offers more dramatic results in tone and texture, reaching deeper layers of skin. After about a week of downtime (you'll look badly sunburned), your natural healing response kicks in, replacing damaged tissue with fresh, younger-looking skin. Cost: around $700.

You want to relieve redness. Immediately, shelve aggressive anti-agers such as retinoid-containing creams and glycolic acid peels.

Nightly, use a cream made with calming botanicals such as licorice extract or feverfew to help control unwanted redness.

Once (4 weeks ahead), if it's in your budget, try a single Intense Pulsed Light session. Experts say you'll average about a 20 percent decrease in diffuse ruddiness after one treatment. Bonus: Because IPL employs several wavelengths of light to remove unwanted pigment, you'll likely see an improvement in brown spots as well. Side effects include mild redness and swelling that subside within a day or two.

WAIT . . . AM I YOUNGER YET?

Science has confirmed that the nutrients in our food can slow down and even reverse aging. And these benefits go way beneath skin deep, to make you younger inside as well as outside. When you eat well, the repair starts immediately on a cellular level, but some benefits take years.

"Certain effects may happen quickly, but it's best to take a long-term perspective when you're trying to change your body," says Tamas Horvath, PhD, a neurobiologist at Yale University.

So when will those antioxidants in your salad start attacking the free radicals ravaging your body? How many fish dinners before you reap the brain-boosting benefits of omega-3s? And how long until that daily vitamin D supplement leads to stronger bones? Here's exactly how and when you can expect the health payoff you want.

In Hours You Can . . .

BEAT STRESS. Vitamin B6 deficiency has been linked to anxiety, stress, and depression, and women are more likely to become deficient in B6 as they age, according to researchers at the Jean Mayer USDA Human Nutrition Research Center on Aging at Tufts University.

"When B6 makes its way to your brain, it facilitates synthesis of neurotransmitters, such as dopamine, which makes you feel calm and happy," says Hanjo Hellmann, PhD, a plant biologist at Washington State University. "But if you have a B6 deficiency, your brain may not be able to make enough dopamine."

The vitamin is found in a variety of foods, but it's especially high in potatoes, bananas, red meat, poultry, and chickpeas. Once eaten, B6 is quickly distributed throughout the body but isn't stored well, so we need a consistent daily supply. Dr. Hellmann recommends getting 1 to 2 milligrams of B6 every day—the amount in about one medium russet potato and a chicken breast—to help you produce enough stress-busting dopamine.

PREVENT CELL DAMAGE THAT CAUSES CANCER. Antioxidants, which are especially abundant in fruits and vegetables, are powerful compounds that cancel out cancer-causing free radicals before they damage cells.

"Antioxidants begin working almost immediately upon absorption—as soon as they find a free radical to interact with," Dr. Hellmann says. But don't think you're set for the week after eating a big salad. Antioxidants remain active for only a few hours and need to be continually replenished. "Plus, they are a diverse group and don't all have the same functions," he says. "The key is always having plenty in your body to take on anything that comes along."

That means eating as much produce as possible and mixing up the types as often as you can.

In 1 Week You Can . . .

LOWER YOUR BLOOD PRESSURE NATURALLY. Potassium supplements are an effective treatment for hypertension, but they can be dangerous for you as you age, according to the American Heart Association.

Scientists at St. George's, University of London found that food sources of potassium are as effective as supplements in fighting high blood pressure—without side effects. The mineral is found in clams and in almost every fruit and vegetable but especially in potatoes, dried peaches, avocados, and bananas. Study participants with high blood pressure ate 3,754 milligrams of potassium per day and lowered their blood pressure to prehypertension levels after just 1 week.

"If you have normal kidneys, you'll use and excrete potassium within hours, which is why getting plenty of fruits and vegetables a day is so important. A steady stream of potassium will control your blood pressure," says Christine Gerbstadt, MD, RD, of the American Dietetic Association. Just be sure to discuss dietary changes with your doctor if you're on blood pressure medications.

In 5 Weeks You Can . . .

BOOST YOUR MEMORY. An Australian study found that folate boosts memory in as little as 35 days. Women who participated in the study, published in the *Journal of Nutrition,* saw improved memory performance after taking 750 micrograms of folate daily. That's about 1 cup of cooked spinach and 1 cup of cooked lentils. Though folate supplements (folic acid) are recommended during pregnancy to

(continued)

help prevent birth defects, you should otherwise get your folate from food, says Dr. Gerbstadt.

In 6 Weeks You Can . . .

LOWER DANGEROUS HOMOCYSTEINE LEVELS. An analysis of 25 studies on B vitamins and homocysteine in the *American Journal of Clinical Nutrition* concluded that taking 800 micrograms of folate supplements daily for 6 to 8 weeks reduces homocysteine concentrations up to 23 percent.

Don't exceed 1,000 micrograms per day, however, or you could trigger symptoms of a B12 deficiency. Good food sources of folate are meat, fish, eggs, and dairy.

In 2 Months You Can . . .

IMPROVE HEART HEALTH. Omega-3s, essential fatty acids in which Americans are known to be deficient, have a wide range of impressive health benefits—from smoothing your skin and aiding weight loss to boosting your mood and minimizing the effects of arthritis. (See Chapter 20: The Vanishing Youth Nutrient.)

However, the ability of omega-3s—found in oily fish (like salmon, mackerel, and anchovies) and in plant sources (flaxseed, walnuts, and spinach)—to prevent heart disease is perhaps best understood. Although some of the heart-health benefits kick in shortly after you digest your salmon, the effects won't last unless you eat these essential fatty acids consistently so that your body reaches a healthy satura-tion level, says Susan Raatz, PhD, RD, an assistant professor of medicine at the Uni-versity of Minnesota: "If you are deficient in omega-3s and begin eating at least two 3-ounce servings of fatty fish a week, your heart will see significant benefits in 4 to 8 weeks."

In 3 Months You Can . . .

FIGHT DEMENTIA. Omega-3s are also crucial to brain health and development, says Stephen Cunnane, PhD, an omega-3 expert at the University of Sherbrooke's

Research Centre on Aging in Quebec. Many studies have found that variations in Alzheimer's disease rates across countries can be predicted by the quantity of fish in the diet.

A study published in *Neuroscience Research* found that patients with mild dementia improved their short-term memory after taking omega-3s daily for 3 months. Another recent study found that depressive feelings in suicidal patients diminished after taking 2.1 grams of omega-3s daily for 3 months. A 3-ounce serving of wild salmon contains nearly 2 grams of omega-3s.

In 1 Year You Can . . .

IMPROVE YOUR VISION. Lutein, a natural plant pigment known as a carotenoid, concentrates in the retina and lens to protect and strengthen your eyes.

"Lutein is important to eye health," says Elizabeth Johnson, PhD, a scientist who studies vision at Tufts University. In a study conducted at North Chicago VA Medical Center, researchers found that patients with age-related macular degeneration improved in multiple measures of vision after taking 12 milligrams of lutein daily for a year.

You can easily get that dose from food, particularly green leafy vegetables such as ½ cup of cooked spinach, Dr. Johnson says. Other top sources of this antioxidant are peas, broccoli, and corn.

BUILD STRONGER BONES. Vitamin D allows your body to absorb the calcium needed to build stronger bones and reduce your risk of osteoporosis. An analysis of multiple vitamin D studies in the *Journal of the American Medical Association* found that a daily supplement of 700 to 800 IU of vitamin D combined with calcium reduces the risk of bone fractures by 26 percent after 2 years. D is found in fortified milk and cereals as well as in fish and eggs, yet supplements are generally accepted as safe.

CHAPTER 28

The ABCs of BEAUTIFUL SKIN

Topical vitamins deliver potent anti-aging benefits right where you need them most. Here are five to start using today.

You might eat your fruits and veggies. You might even pop a multi every day. Yet your skin is still missing out on the value of vitamins. Research shows that these nutrients are essential for preventing and reversing many signs of aging.

A well-balanced diet is important, of course. Eating a variety of healthy foods helps keep skin supple and glowing.

But the fact is, "the body delivers only a certain percentage of vitamins to your skin, no matter how much you ingest," says Mary Lupo, MD, New Orleans dermatologist and clinical professor of dermatology at Tulane University School of Medicine. Plus, there's no way to send them straight to your crow's feet or brown spots. The solution: applying vitamins topically to deliver maximum benefits—everything from improving texture and tone to fading under-eye circles. Follow this user's guide to the letter, and soon your skin will look better than ever.

VITAMIN A: BEST OVERALL AGE FIGHTER

Find it in OTC lotions, night creams (vitamin A derivatives are known as retinoids), and prescription products.

Vitamin A has been proven to reduce wrinkles, fade brown spots, and smooth roughness.

"There are more than 700 published studies on retinoids—they're tried-and-true ingredients. Anyone who wants younger-looking skin should use one," says Doris Day, MD, assistant clinical professor of dermatology at New York University Langone Medical Center.

How to use: Apply your retinoid at night because sunlight inactivates most forms of vitamin A. Prescription retinoids work fastest, within 4 to 8 weeks. The downside: They're irritating, causing redness, scaling, and flaking that last for weeks or longer. OTC products are best for beginners; you'll experience fewer side effects because the retinol they contain is slowly converted to retinoic acid, the active ingredient in prescription creams. To avoid irritation, apply an OTC or prescription retinoid every second or third night, at least for the first 2 weeks, and build up to nightly use. Apply sparingly; a pea-size amount is enough to cover your entire face.

Try: Neutrogena Dermatologics Retinol NX Serum ($72, www. qvc.com) or RoC Multi-Correxion Night Treatment ($25, drugstores). If your skin is sensitive, two new retinoids are particularly gentle. Clinical studies show that retinyl propionate, available in Olay Professional Pro-X Deep Wrinkle Treatment ($40, drugstores), significantly improves skin after 12 weeks without being as drying as the more potent retinol. Ready to trade up to a prescription retinoid? Ask about Atralin (about $150), which contains two potent emollients. "Even my most sensitive patients are able to tolerate it," says Dr. Day.

VITAMIN B3: BOOSTS HYDRATION TO REDUCE REDNESS

Find it in lotions, creams, and serums. It's often called niacinamide on the label.

Proven to increase production of ceramides and fatty acids, two key components of your skin's outer protective barrier.

"As that barrier is strengthened, skin is better able to keep moisture in and

THREE NEW AGE-DEFYING ANTIOXIDANTS

These skin protectors might be hard to pronounce, but they are powerful anti-agers. Here we dig up the science behind these top defenders.

Phloretin

Found in SkinCeuticals Phloretin CF ($152, www. skinceuticals.com), fades sun spots.

RESEARCH: In one study using this serum, 62 percent of women saw a significant lightening of brown spots after 8 weeks.

Pyratine

Found in Pyratine-6 Lotion ($86, radiantskinclinic.com), fights fine lines.

RESEARCH: Users noted a 28 percent improvement in wrinkles after 12 weeks of use, say researchers at the University of California, Irvine.

Astaxanthin

Found in DermaE Age-Defying Night Creme ($37, drugstore.com), reduces inflammation.

RESEARCH: In a clinical study, an astaxanthin cream diminished puffiness. Bonus: It also increased moisture and firmness.

irritants out—making B3 a great ingredient if your complexion is dry or sensitive," says Leslie Baumann, MD, director of the Division of Cosmetic Dermatology, University of Miami. In one study, a moisturizer with niacinamide improved the flushing and blushing of rosacea, a common condition that can worsen with age. Another B3 benefit: It inhibits the transfer of pigment to skin cells, minimizing dark spots.

How to use: For maximum results, apply B3 in the morning and evening. To reduce irritation from your retinoid, use it in conjunction with niacinamide. "Mix them together in the palm of your hand before applying. They won't inactivate each other," says Dr. Baumann. Besides decreasing side effects, the combo produces superior anti-aging benefits.

Try: La Roche-Posay Rosaliac Anti-Redness Moisturizer ($34, CVS) or Olay Regenerist Micro-Sculpting Cream ($22, drugstores).

VITAMIN C: ALL-AROUND ANTI-AGER

Find it in moisturizers formulated to keep vitamin C stable (opaque, airtight containers are ideal). Look for vitamin C near the middle of the ingredients panel to help ensure the 5 percent or higher concentration needed to see benefits, advises Hema Sundaram, MD, a dermatologist in the Washington, DC, area.

Proven to mop up the free radicals that trigger wrinkling, sagging, and other aging changes. Vitamin C also helps smooth and firm skin and fade brown spots. In one study, women who treated sun-damaged skin with a vitamin C cream for 6 months saw significant improvement in fine lines and discoloration. Though the benefits of retinoids (see vitamin A) and vitamin C sound similar, using both delivers more complexion perfection.

"Skin aging occurs in various ways, so you need multiple forms of defense and repair," says Dr. Lupo.

How to use: Apply vitamin C in the morning before sunscreen to shield your skin from any UV-generated free radicals that get past your sunblock.

Try: SkinMedica Vitamin C + E Complex ($90, www. skinmedica.com) or Avalon Organics Vitamin C Renewal Facial Cream ($21, avalonorganics. com). These products contain ascorbic acid or magnesium ascorbyl phosphate (the skin-friendliest forms of vitamin C) in combination with vitamin E (it's listed as alpha-tocopherol or tocopherol acetate). This duo provides 4 times more protection against free radicals when applied together.

VITAMIN E: EASES DRYNESS AND BOLSTERS SKIN'S UV DEFENSE

Find it in sunscreens and after-sun products. The best products contain at least 1 percent vitamin E, so it will be listed near the middle of the ingredients panel.

Proven to quell dryness by helping skin retain its natural moisturizers. Also, vitamin E's potent ability to neutralize damaging free radicals has earned it the moniker "the protector." A slew of studies document its superstar status. In one, vitamin E significantly reduced the number of these unstable molecules created after exposure to cigarette smoke. Others show that when it's used before UV exposure, skin is less red, swollen, and dry.

How to use: Apply before and after serious sun exposure. A single strong blast of UV light can destroy half the skin's natural supply of vitamin E, so shore up defenses by slathering on a sunscreen supplemented with E and C before going into the sun—the C helps ensure effectiveness. An after-sun salve with vitamin E helps, too, says Oceanside, California, dermatologist Jens Thiele, MD, PhD, a vitamin E expert. Some studies show that the anti-inflammatory action kicks in to reduce damage even after you've been in the sun.

Try: Neutrogena Age Shield Face Sunblock SPF 55 ($8, www. drugstore. com), Dr Dennis Gross Skincare Powerful Sun Protection SPF 30 Daily Sunscreen Towelettes ($18, sephora.com), Clinique After-Sun Rescue Balm with Aloe ($20, clinique.com), or Hawaiian Tropic After Sun Body Butter ($8, drugstores).

VITAMIN K: FOR YOUNGER, BRIGHTER EYES

Find it in eye creams that also contain retinol.

Proven to possibly help lighten under-eye circles. Fragile capillaries that allow blood to leak into skin are considered one cause of under-eye circles, and vitamin K (aka phytonadione) may put the skids on this seepage by controlling blood clotting. Daily use of a vitamin K cream significantly lightened circles after 4 months in one study, but because the cream also contained retinol, researchers aren't sure which ingredient deserves credit for the improvement. Retinol alone thickens the translucent under-eye skin (making it harder to see the dark blood vessels below) and lightens melanin that makes circles more prominent. Still, it can't hurt to try a cream that contains vitamin K and retinol. According to Dr. Baumann, the retinol may enhance vitamin K's ability to penetrate skin and knock out darkness.

How to use: Apply nightly. First allow skin to become acclimated to the retinol—use once or twice the first week, and add a night every week after.

Try: NeoStrata Bionic Eye Cream ($50, www. neostrata.com), Quintessence Skin Science Clarifying Under-Eye Serum ($67, www. baumannstore.com), or Jan Marini Factor-A Eyes for Dark Circles ($78, www. myjanmarini.com).

PREVENTION'S DEFY-YOUR-AGE BEAUTY AWARDS

We subjected the leading anti-aging products to rigorous testing and emerged with seven that really, truly deliver visible results. Meet the winners—and watch wrinkles, brown spots, and other over-40 skin issues disappear!

They say you get what you pay for, but our beauty awards this year prove real skin care stars can erase years and be budget-friendly. Each winner costs less than $50 and hits the anti-aging jackpot. We know this because we found out which anti-agers live up to their claims. Here's how it works: Each product (35 in all!) was used by five women over age 40 for up to 8 weeks. A dermatologist then analyzed their skin; the facial products were evaluated with state-of-the-art equipment like the Visia Complexion Analysis system, which takes and compares before-and-after photos to detect improvement. If you're yearning to look younger, prepare to fall for these top picks.

Best Day Lotion with SPF

Olay Professional Pro-X Age Repair Lotion with SPF 30 ($47, drugstores)

Wrinkles, meet your match. This luxurious lotion packs two powerful peptides that work to smooth fine lines and firm skin by speeding the production of new collagen. Testers also noticed (or should we say didn't notice?) fewer brown spots, thanks to niacinamide, a B vitamin that has the bonus benefit of increasing hydration—a plus for those with dry, sensitive skin, says judge Susan Weinkle, MD. Sunscreenphobes, rejoice: Though it's packed with a broad-spectrum SPF 30, Florida testers loved how the lotion seeped quickly into skin without feeling heavy or tacky.

USE IT RIGHT: Slather on exposed areas at least 20 minutes before heading out the door. To ensure protection, allow it to soak in before putting on your makeup.

Best Night Cream

RoC Multi-Correxion Night Treatment ($25, drugstores)

After 2 weeks, testers were hooked on this dream cream: "My skin seemed to glow in the morning," says one. By week 8, judge David Bank, MD, reported significant improvement in fine lines and brown spots—as many as 10 spots on each tester faded away. He credits proven multitaskers like retinol and vitamin C, which rev radiance, smooth and firm skin, and lighten discoloration. Though both ingredients can be irritating, testers didn't experience any side effects. They did report that the cream left their skin feeling soft all day, thanks to glycerin and vitamin E.

USE IT RIGHT: Apply a small amount to face and neck at night—ideally, 20 minutes before bedtime to maximize absorption. To avoid diluting its effectiveness, don't use with any other leave-on products.

Best Lip Treatment

Lancome L'Absolu Rouge La Base Revitalizing Lip Treatment SPF 10 ($29, www.lancome-usa.com)

This elegant balm does more than leave lips smooth and supple. It plumps them up and gives fine lines the kiss-off! Testers reported that lips immediately looked fuller for up to 3 hours, and even longer with continued use. The workhorse ingredient is Pro-Xylane, a sugar molecule that boosts production of collagen and skin's built-in moisturizers, says judge David Goldberg, MD.

USE IT RIGHT: Apply throughout the day, allowing it to sink in before putting on gloss or lipstick.

Best Microdermabrasion Treatment

Estée Lauder Idealist Dual-Action Refinishing Treatment ($49.50, www.esteelauder.com)

Ready to get your glow on? This skin polisher instantly boosts brightness, making it a great pick-me-up before an important event. But the real anti-aging benefits came from regular use: After just 1 month of weekly application, judge Mary Lupo, MD, detected that testers' pores were smaller, fine lines were smoother, and skin was more radiant. That's thanks to salicylic acid, glucosamine, and a blend of spherical beads that slough away dulling dead cells and dislodge debris that can trigger breakouts. Prone to irritation? Dr. Lupo gives this ultragentle moisturizing formula the thumbs-up even for sensitive skin.

(continued)

USE IT RIGHT: Rub onto clean damp skin to activate the soothing warmth, which improves penetration; rinse after 5 minutes. Apply weekly at first (if using a retinoid, wait until skin adapts to it); increase to several times a week as skin becomes acclimated.

Best Adult Acne Treatment

Avon Clearskin Professional Acne Treatment System ($32, avon.com)

This easy-to-use system scored an A+ for beating blemishes. "Testers reported improvement within just a few weeks," says judge Macrene Alexiades-Armenakas, MD. But unlike teenagers' treatments, which often dry out 40-plus complexions and make wrinkles more pronounced, this trio of products—a scrub, a toner, and an oil-free lotion—contains humectants that soften and smooth. The regimen relies on salicylic acid, which kills bacteria, dries oil, and unclogs pores, to eradicate existing pimples and prevent new ones. Meanwhile, it speeds skin turnover and stimulates collagen production, so you can forget about fine lines, too.

USE IT RIGHT: Start by using the system once a day, then gradually increase to twice a day, if needed.

Best Hand Cream

Neutrogena Norwegian Formula Age Shield Hand Cream SPF 30 ($6, drugstores)

Talk about a hands-down winner! Testers gave this velvety-smooth cream high marks for providing all-day hydration that left even the driest skin soft and supple without feeling greasy. Judge Ranella Hirsch, MD, chalks up the improvement to heavy-duty humectants and emollients that attract and trap water into skin, smoothing fine lines and wrinkles. Potent UV protection helps keep future damage off your hands. The best evidence of all: Each tester said she'd buy it.

USE IT RIGHT: Apply every morning and after each hand washing. It's concentrated, so you need only a dab.

Best Eye Cream

Skin Effects by Dr. Jeffrey Dover Cell2Cell Anti-Aging Eye Treatment ($15, CVS pharmacy)

If you're seeing crow's feet and dark circles, you'll want to keep this eye cream in your sights. Made with peptides and dermaxyl, a nonirritating synthetic retinoid, it significantly decreased crinkles, brown spots, and under-eye darkness in testers, minus any redness or peeling, reports judge Tina Alster, MD. Moisture magnets such as hyaluronic acid attract water to this thin, often dry skin, making it look youthfully plump. Makeup lovers sang its praises: "I got away with wearing less concealer," says one tester. "It absorbed so quickly, I didn't have to wait to apply my eye shadow," says another. Even better, makeup didn't slip and slide.

USE IT RIGHT: Gently apply a pea-size drop in the morning and evening. "Aggressive rubbing can cause irritation and wrinkling," says Dr. Alster. Follow with a broad-spectrum SPF 30 in the morning to protect fresh cells.

Meet Our Judges

Macrene Alexiades-Armenakas, MD, assistant clinical professor at Yale University School of Medicine; practices in New York City

Tina Alster, MD, clinical professor at Georgetown University; practices in Washington, DC

David Bank, MD, associate professor at Columbia University/Presbyterian Hospital; practices in Mt. Kisco, New York

David Goldberg, MD, clinical professor at Mount Sinai School of Medicine; practices in New York, New Jersey, and Florida

Ranella Hirsch, MD, past president of the American Society of Cosmetic Dermatology & Aesthetic Surgery; practices in Cambridge, Massachusetts

Mary Lupo, MD, clinical professor at Tulane University School of Medicine; practices in New Orleans

Susan Weinkle, MD, assistant clinical professor at the University of South Florida; practices in Bradenton, Florida

CHAPTER 29

AGELESS
Beauty

*21 fast, easy ways to look young—
and stay that way*

Planning some fun in the sun? Whether summer is approaching or you're going on a sun-drenched vacation, it's a real treat to lighten your beauty routine: ditching your foundation and blush for a simple swipe of bronzer; letting your locks succumb to their natural waves. The flip side to going a bit more natural is the number it can do on your looks.

"Harmful UV rays are the most obvious culprit in causing wrinkles and brown spots, but they can also make your skin and hair appear dry, so you look older than your years," says dermatologist David H. McDaniel, MD, director of the Institute of Anti-Aging Research in Virginia Beach, Virginia.

We talked to leading dermatologists and dug through a mountain of research and products to offer natural, easy, schedule-friendly tips guaranteed to keep every part of you looking gorgeous and young.

Try a sun protection pill. Aside from daily use of a broad-spectrum SPF 30 sunscreen, boost your UV protection by taking an antioxidant supplement such as Heliocare ($60 for 60, www. drugstore.com) or SunPill ($20 for 30, www. sunpill.com). New research from the University of Miami School of Medicine shows that the fern extract in these pills significantly reduced UVA-related DNA damage that leads to wrinkling and brown spots. For best results, pop one each day starting a week before you plan on fun in the sun.

"This allows the antioxidants to build up in your system for maximum protection," says Leslie Baumann, MD, director of the University of Miami Division of Cosmetic Dermatology.

Exfoliate the smart way. Alternate between daily use of chemical and mechanical exfoliation. This does a better job of removing the dead cells that build up more on the skin's surface in the summer, which leaves a radiant glow, says Debra Jaliman, MD, an assistant professor of dermatology at Mount Sinai School of Medicine. Switch between using an alpha hydroxy acid (AHA) lotion and a Buf-Puf or scrubbing granules.

Layer lip balm with SPF. Slick on a formula with a built-in SPF of at least 15 underneath even an SPF-containing lipstick or gloss to further guard against thinning, dryness, and sun spots.

"Lips lack a protective outer layer, so they're incredibly sensitive to UV rays," says Dr. Baumann.

Use sunscreen to protect hair in a pinch. Going swimming? Comb your regular sunscreen through your strands; this forms a barrier that prevents chlorine and salt water from stripping your color and drying out hair, explains Los Angeles hairstylist Jessica Galván.

Try a caffeine-packed àpres sun treatment. A topical jolt of caffeine significantly reduces UV-induced roughness and wrinkling in mice, according to one study. A more recent finding shows it might even help curb skin cancer by suppressing ATR, a protein that enables precancerous cells to survive and replicate. The research is preliminary, but applying a cream that contains about 1 percent caffeine after sun exposure couldn't hurt.

Try: Topix Replenix CF Anti-Photoaging Complex SPF 45 ($35, www. skinstore.com).

Boost post-sun hydration. Reduce UV-induced dryness from sun exposure by slathering clean skin with moisturizer and covering with a warm, damp towel for 5 minutes.

"The heat activates the lotion's ingredients, which keeps skin supple," says Mary P. Lupo, MD, New Orleans dermatologist and clinical professor of dermatology at Tulane University School of Medicine.

Save your self-tan. Steer clear of exfoliating scrubs and creams that contain retinol and AHA for a few days after using your self-tanner.

"These products slough the top layer of skin, removing color in the process," says Natalie Cupid, senior technician and manager of Sundara Airbrush Tanning in New York City.

Strengthen nails with a supplement. Take 2.5 milligrams of the B vitamin biotin daily.

"This supplement helps prevent breakage from too much exposure to salt and chlorine," says Jin Soon Choi, owner of Jin Soon Natural Hand and Foot Spas. Research shows that a daily dose of the nutrient increases nail thickness by 25 percent, making nails less apt to split and tear.

Get a smoother shave. Wait at least 3 minutes after getting in the shower before you whip out your razor.

"Warm water softens the hair shaft, allowing for a closer cut and longer-lasting smoothness without nicking skin," says Diane Wood, master barber for King of Shaves.

Get younger hands with moisturizer. During the day, use a hand cream containing the lightener kojic acid to soften brown spots. Try Hollywood Hands Professional Anti-Aging Hand Treatment ($16, drugstores). At night, apply a hand cream that contains skin-firming retinol, suggests Dr. Baumann. Try Sally Hansen Age Correct Retinol Hand Cream ($6.50, drugstores). Be sure to wear a sunblock with an SPF of at least 15 as well; these ingredients make skin sensitive.

Wear sandals to keep soles soft. It's tempting this time of year, but avoid walking barefoot—even in the house or on the beach.

"The added pressure causes painful and unsightly calluses to build up," explains Allison Tangorra, a nail artist at DePasquale the Spa in Morris Plains, New Jersey.

Spot treat pimples with a cotton swab. When applying benzoyl peroxide to blemishes, use the tip of a cotton swab to precisely dab it on. This prevents the medication from stripping your self-tanner, says Nicole Weigand, spa director at the Beverly Hills Hotel Spa by La Prairie.

Mop your hairline after wearing a hat. Increased oils can get trapped underneath hats and headbands, causing acne along your forehead, says Cheryl Karcher, MD, a New York dermatologist. Run an antibacterial wipe along your forehead to prevent pimples.

Shampoo with baking soda to remove smog. Higher summertime pollution means more free radicals to zap the shine and color from hair. To remove dulling residue, add a pinch of baking soda to your regular shampoo instead of using a harsh clarifying cleanser.

"It rinses out chemicals without stripping color," says Galván. Bonus: This trick helps prevent discoloration caused by chlorine and salt water, too.

Sleep on a silk pillowcase. "The satiny texture prevents friction from roughing up the cuticle and making hair vulnerable to warm weather–induced frizz," says James Corbett, owner of James Corbett Studio in New York City. If you're really ambitious, wrap your hair in a silk scarf before going to bed.

Self-tan from head to toe. To look longer and leaner, apply self-tanner everywhere, says Dera Enochson, creator of Xen-Tan, a company that makes self-tanners.

"A uniform color helps elongate, but focusing just on your legs or arms can make you look shorter and stockier."

Unclog pores with papaya. Mash up fresh papaya and apply to clean skin for 3 minutes.

→ PREVENTION Alert!

THE YOUTHFUL BONUS OF BLUSH

Women with a vibrant flush are considered more physically attractive by others, according to recent research from the University of St. Andrews in Scotland. With age, blood supply to the skin decreases, causing dullness, says David Colbert, MD, a cosmetic dermatologist in New York City. This is easily corrected with makeup and nightly use of a wrinkle-fighting retinoid cream, which boosts blood supply and oxygen content to skin, restoring a rosy glow.

"This summertime fruit contains enzymes that slough pore-clogging dead cells, leaving skin soft and radiant," says Dr. Karcher.

Choose metal-free hair bands. Avoid ponytail holders that are joined with a small metal bar: They can snag hair and cause split ends, especially when hair is wet and weaker after swimming, explains Rick Mahoney, senior stylist at Devachan Salon in New York City. Instead, look for ties covered entirely with snagproof fabric. Try Goody Ouchless Extra Thick Elastics ($3.50 drugstores).

Use a makeup brush to boost hair shine. Shine products help restore lost moisture and luminosity from increased sun exposure and hotter temps, but many contain heavy silicones that can weigh hair down. The solution? Spritz shine spray onto your blush brush and then sweep over hair.

"The soft bristles help to apply precise, targeted shine without weighing down hair," says Antoinette Beenders, vice president of global creative at Aveda.

Exfoliate heels in the shower. Maximize results for smooth, sexy feet by using a pumice stone on calluses and rough spots at the end of your shower.

"The extra time in the water softens dead cells and makes them easier to remove," says Choi.

Prep your razor. To extend the life of your razor a few days and ensure a smoother shave, drizzle some olive oil on the blade, suggests Cindy Barshop, owner of Completely Bare in New York City.

"The oil prevents rust and product buildup, which can cause nicks."

CHAPTER 30

HAIR COLOR
That Lasts

Here are 12 ways to save money and stretch out time between dye jobs.

Coloring your hair makes you look younger, brighter, and sexier, but it can also be costly and time-consuming.

"Silver strands are porous, so they require more frequent touch-ups than naturally pigmented hair does," says Jason Backe, Clairol's color director and co-owner of the Ted Gibson Salon in New York City. Then there's the issue of roots: Even if you're not fully gray, within a few weeks an obvious line of demarcation can spoil the whole look. Whether you're a do-it-yourself dyer or you have your colorist on speed dial, use our expert tips to save cash and spread out time between coloring sessions.

LIGHT-AS-AIR HAIR CARE

Conditioner is essential for silky, tangle-free hair, but it often has heavy softening agents that weigh strands down. To the rescue: a new generation of products made with "terminal amino silicones." According to Pantene scientist Teca Gillespie, these silicone particles maintain volume more efficiently while still detangling so hair stays manageable. Try: Pantene Pro-V Beautiful Lengths Conditioner ($8.99, www. drugstore.com) and Ion Extreme Moisture Creme ($7.50, www. sallybeauty.com).

BEFORE YOU COLOR

Wash with a clarifying shampoo a day prior to dyeing. "Stronger detergents remove excess product buildup, so color penetrates deeper and lasts longer," explains Eva Scrivo, the owner of Eva Scrivo Salon in New York City.

Choose fade-resistant shades such as blonde or brunette. "Reds wash away a week or two faster because they contain smaller color molecules, which escape from hair more easily," says Karla Siereveld, PhD, a scientist at Procter & Gamble. Bonus: These tones flatter over-40 faces.

Pick the right formula. Demipermanents (like Clairol Natural Instincts; $9, drugstores) last for up to 28 shampoos, and permanent colors (like Garnier 100% Color Vibrant Colors by Nutrisse; $8, drugstores) don't rinse out but fade over time. Highlights—from a pro or an at-home kit such as Revlon Custom Effects Highlights ($11; drugstores)—buy you the most time: "There's a less obvious line, so roots aren't as noticeable," says Lorri Goddard-Clark, author of *The Hair Color Mix Book.*

AFTER YOU COLOR

Wait 48 hours to shampoo. "Dye molecules need time to set into strands," explains Scrivo.

53

THE PERCENTAGE OF WOMEN WHO SPEND MORE TIME MANAGING THEIR FRIZZ THAN THEY DO EXERCISING, ACCORDING TO P&G

Cleanse with a shampoo for color-treated hair, which contains gentler detergents, and rinse with tepid water. "Hot water expands the cuticle, contributing to fading," says Scrivo.

Install a showerhead water purifier. "Tap water contains chlorine, which is a bleaching agent," explains Goddard-Clark. "Even well water has minerals like copper that coat the hair and alter its hue." Try the iWater Shower Purification System ($50, myiwater.com).

Use a conditioner or styling aid with built-in sunscreens to prevent the sun from stripping your shade. Try Redken Color Extend Conditioner ($14; redken.com for salons); UV filters bind to safeguard strands.

Spritz on a thermal protection spray such as Dove Heat Defense Therapy Mist ($5; drugstores) before styling. Polymers prevent heat from penetrating hair and breaking down the dye molecules.

72-HOUR FRESH-HAIR SECRET

Blow-drying can strip your color and dry out strands, says Marcos Diaz, a session stylist at Ion Studio in NYC. Follow these tips to keep your locks looking lovely:

DAY 1: Shampoo twice in a row with a mild product to remove residue that weighs hair down; then condition only the ends.

DAY 2: Spritz a dry shampoo onto your roots; the powder formula absorbs existing oil and prevents more from building up.

DAY 3: Switch your part to boost volume and hide less-than-squeaky-clean roots; touch up with your blow-dryer to restore bounce.

Switch to an ionic blow-dryer, which has tourmaline, a type of stone that generates negative ions that reduce frizz and cut dulling dryingtime in half.

ON A REGULAR BASIS

Apply a conditioning mask once weekly. The added hydration strengthens strands, making them less prone to environmental damage that causes fading. Also, creating a smooth surface helps hair better reflect light, making color look more vibrant. Love your locks with these great products.

Prevent fading. Semipermanent dyes in Ken Paves Healthy Hair Boost Up Color Drops ($40, www. ulta.com) renew your shade when added to conditioner or styling products; choose from 6 colors.

Beat brassiness. Antioxidants and sunscreens in Pureology InCharge Plus Firm Finishing Spray ($20, pureology.com for salons) prevent dulling UV damage.

Boost shine. The silicones in Frédéric Fekkai Salon Glaze Clear Shine Rinse ($28, sephora.com) rejuvenate radiance.

Perk up highlights. Brightening honey, caramel, and wheat germ in John Frieda Sheer Blonde Highlight Activating Shampoo ($6.50, drugstores) bring out lighter streaks; also available for brunettes.

72

THE PERCENTAGE OF WOMEN WHO HAVE MORE SPRING IN THEIR STEP ON GOOD HAIR DAYS, ACCORDING TO TRESEMMÉ

Disguise stray grays. With a messproof mascara wand and a peroxide-free formula, Avon Advance Techniques Color Protection Grey Root Touch-Up ($5, avon.com) hides silver strands until you shampoo.

Three weeks postcoloring, switch to a color-enhancing shampoo every other time you wash. Available in shades ranging from light blonde to dark brunette, these formulas contain ingredients like cocoa beans and sunflower seed extract that brighten your hue and subtly disguise grays.

Monthly, use an at-home glaze or gloss (available in clear and tinted formulas) to add high-wattage shine and intensify a fading shade. "It's akin to putting a topcoat of polish on your hair," says Backe.

AGELESS HAIRSTYLE: THE PONYTAIL

You know it's fast and easy, but this insta-style is also an insta-youth boost. "Pulling hair back focuses attention on your cheekbones and gives your face a lift," says Nunzio Saviano, a senior stylist at the Oscar Blandi Salon in New York City.

FOR DAY: Casually sweep hair softly, and secure it at the nape of the neck.

FOR NIGHT: Pull hair smooth and higher at the crown; free a small strand and wrap it around your band (fasten with a bobby pin) for an elegant finish.

CHAPTER 31

FINALLY!
Sunscreens You'll
LOVE TO WEAR

Whatever your complaint about UV protectors,
we've got you covered.

Despite elegant new formulations and innovative packaging that makes sunscreen application a snap, too much skin is still going uncovered. In a 2008 survey by Coppertone, nearly half of respondents admitted they didn't wear sunscreen at all. Until now, that is. Prepare to excuseproof your sunscreen use!

EXCUSE: "SUNSCREEN MAKES ME BREAK OUT"

The truth: Fear of aggravating acne is the number-one reason women shun sunscreen, says Robert A. Weiss, MD, immediate past president of the American Society for Dermatologic Surgery. But guess what? Protecting skin from UV light curtails future breakouts.

"The sun stimulates oil glands and thickens skin, so pores become blocked," explains Dr. Weiss.

SUNSCREEN ALERT: PROTECT THESE PARTS, TOO

Any area exposed to sunlight is at risk of UV damage, says Amy Wechsler, MD, New York City dermatologist and psychiatrist and author of *The Mind-Beauty Connection.* Here's how to age-proof three frequently forgotten spots.

Scalp

The sun can penetrate hair, putting you at risk of hidden melanoma over time.

PROTECT IT: Spritz on an SPF styling product before hitting the beach. Try Frédéric Fekkai Coiff Defense Pre-Style Thermal/UV Protectant ($25, sephora.com). Wear a tightly woven hat for extra insurance.

Ears

The rims of the ears are so often missed they've become the primary places for basal or squamous-cell carcinoma, which are the two most common types of skin cancer, reports the Skin Cancer Foundation.

PROTECT THEM: Apply your sunscreen here first so it becomes a habit.

Nails

Sun exposure breaks down proteins in the nail, causing vertical ridges.

PROTECT THEM: Apply a UV-absorbing topcoat, or rub on hand cream containing SPF. Try Barielle Ultra Speed Dry Manicure Extender ($16, www. barielle.com).

54

THE PERCENTAGE OF AMERICANS WHO GOT SUNBURNED IN THE LAST 3 YEARS. PROTECT YOUR SKIN BY APPLYING SUNSCREEN HEAD TO TOE 20 MINUTES BEFORE GOING OUTDOORS

Problem solver: Keep breakouts at bay with a lightweight, nonoily lotion like Coppertone NutraShield Faces 70+ SPF with Dual Defense ($10.50, drugstores), which is proven not to clog pores.

EXCUSE: "IT'S MESSY TO REAPPLY SUNSCREEN OVER MAKEUP"

The truth: Not freshening your sunscreen is akin to committing skin suicide. Here's why: The potency of sunscreen decreases after just a couple of hours, and a mere 10 minutes of daily exposure to aging UVA rays is known to cause changes that lead to wrinkles and brown spots within a few months.

Problem solver: A brush-on tinted mineral sunscreen powder such as bareMinerals SPF 30 Natural Sunscreen ($28, bareescentuals.com) is perfect for quick touch-ups before dashing out to lunch or running errands midday. Besides helping to even out your skin tone, the minerals naturally diffuse light, so your complexion looks smoother and more luminous.

EXCUSE: "I SWEAT IT OFF SO QUICKLY"

The truth: This lament, common among outdoor athletes, has merit: Sweating decreases the effectiveness of sunscreen, and so does wiping the skin to remove the sweat, says James Spencer, MD, associate clinical professor of dermatology at Mount Sinai School of Medicine. Look for a sport sunscreen labeled very water resistant or very water/sweat resistant. That means it's proven to protect for 80 minutes. Still, to be safe, reapply often.

Problem solver: In addition to being very water/sweat resistant, Banana

SURPRISING BLEMISH BUSTER: SUNSCREEN

UV rays trigger sebaceous glands to pump out 26 percent more of the oil that causes acne, putting you at risk of breakouts, according to new research from Vichy skin care brand. A broad-spectrum sunscreen blocks these rays. One for over-40, pimple-prone skin: Aveeno Positively Radiant Tinted Moisturizer with SPF 30 ($17, drugstores), which is oil-free and contains soy to fade brown spots.

Boat UltraMist Sport Performance Continuous Spray SPF 85 ($11.50, drugstores) sprays on clear, so hands don't get greasy rubbing it in (a boon for golf and tennis players). A nozzle that works at any angle makes coating hard-to-reach places a breeze.

EXCUSE: "MY SKIN IS SENSITIVE"

The truth: Chemical sunscreens, which absorb UV light, can be irritating. Instead, opt for a physical sunblock that reflects UV rays; these products contain zinc oxide or titanium dioxide, which rarely upset sensitive skin. Even better, because sunblocks don't allow skin to get as hot as sunscreens do, they're less likely to aggravate redness from conditions such as rosacea, says Dr. Weiss.

Problem solver: Some sunblocks create a whitish cast, but the ultrafine zinc and titanium in Neutrogena Sensitive Skin Sunblock Lotion SPF 60+ with PureScreen ($11, drugstores) quickly vanish into skin. It's also fragrance-free, further reducing the chance of irritation.

EXCUSE: "SUNSCREEN MAKES MY FACE SHINY"

The truth: Even some oil-free formulas leave skin looking (and feeling) like a grease slick. They're often too heavy to apply under makeup as well. As a result, many women rely on the SPF in makeup, a habit worth breaking: A

WHAT'S YOUR MELANOMA RISK?

A new study found six factors that significantly raise the risk of melanoma, the deadliest form of skin cancer. The disease is curable when spotted early. The 5-year survival rate is now more than 90 percent.

Melanoma Risk Factors	Yes	No
1. Outdoor summer jobs for 3 or more years as a teen	___	___
2. Blistering sunburns as a teen	___	___
3. Red or blonde hair	___	___
4. Freckling of the upper back	___	___
5. Family history	___	___
6. History of actinic keratoses	___	___

Answer Key

ONE YES: 2 to 3 times normal risk.

PROTECT YOURSELF: Be vigilant about self-checks, and see a dermatologist for an annual exam. Wear sunscreen (at least SPF 30) every day.

TWO YESES: 5 to 10 times normal risk.

PROTECT YOURSELF: Stay in the shade during the sun's strongest hours—10 a.m. to 4 p.m.—and wear a hat and pants when you can, in addition to the tips here.

THREE OR MORE YESES: 10 to 20 times normal risk.

PROTECT YOURSELF: See a dermatologist at least twice a year for full-body skin checks, in addition to the above tips.

study did show that even under typical office or home conditions, foundation can shift and wear off after a few hours.

Problem solver: Thanks to its ultra-airy texture, La Roche-Posay Anthelios 60 Ultra Light Sunscreen Fluid for Face ($27.50, CVS) absorbs quickly and dries to a matte finish, so foundation glides on smoothly and doesn't slide off. Skip-a-step bonus: It's moisturizing, so you don't need a separate day cream.

EXCUSE: "IT'S TOO LATE; THE DAMAGE IS ALREADY DONE"

The truth: If you still think most sun damage occurs before you hit age 20, here's news: You get less than 25 percent of your total sun exposure by age 18, not the 80 percent experts used to believe. In fact, by age 40, you've soaked up only about half your total lifetime exposure. And no matter what your age, daily sunscreen use reduces damage and allows skin to repair itself, says Dr. Weiss.

Problem solver: Protect skin and boost its natural repair abilities with NIA24 Sun Damage Prevention 100% Mineral Sunscreen SPF 30 ($45, nia24.com). It contains Pro-Niacin, a form of vitamin B3 that helps erase past sun sins by improving skin hydration and minimizing dark spots.

SPECIAL REPORT: SUNSCREENS UNDER FIRE

You apply sunscreen to protect your skin, not harm it, right? But controversies about its safety continue to rage. Here's what is true, and why sunscreens—which are proven to prevent skin cancer and slow signs of aging—are still the best way to keep your skin safe year-round.

Concern: Sunscreens don't protect enough against "aging" UVA rays

Background: In this case, the fears are founded. In a recent study of 13 popular sunscreens, only 5 offered a high degree of UVA protection (though not the highest possible amount); the majority yielded only a medium level. Those are scary findings, considering that UVA accounts for more than 95 percent of the UV rays we're exposed to and triggers far more free radicals that lead to wrinkles and brown spots.

The bottom line: To get the best UVA protection, you have to be a real label hawk. Keep an eye out for these ingredients: avobenzone, Mexoryl, and zinc oxide. To be sure that avobenzone has staying power (ironically, the sun quickly renders it ineffective), it should be paired with stabilizers like octocrylene, Polyester-8, butyloctyl salicylate, or ethylhexyl methoxycrylene. (Helioplex, which is available in Neutrogena sunscreens, is a stabilized form of avobenzone.)

To guard against free radicals, choose sunscreens that contain antioxidants like vitamins C (aka ascorbic acid) and E (aka tocopherol), which reduce these dangerous molecules by as much as 74 percent. The higher up they're listed on the ingredient panel, the greater the concentration.

Concern: They contain ingredients that raise your risk of breast cancer

Background: A popular ingredient in sunscreens, oxybenzone (aka benzophenone-3) has the unique ability to protect against both short UVA rays and the entire UVB spectrum. But consumer groups like the Environmental Working Group (EWG) have questioned its use because a few studies suggested the chemical mimics the effects of estrogen—potentially causing cancer cells to grow more rapidly.

In another study, volunteers applied highly concentrated oxybenzone-containing sunscreens all over their bodies every day for 4 days. Although the oxybenzone absorbed into their bloodstreams, it had no impact on reproductive hormones, including estrogen.

Much ado has also been made of the fact that oxybenzone—which is in everything from cosmetics to food—showed up in trace amounts in 97 percent of urine samples analyzed by the CDC.

But "that doesn't mean it causes an adverse health effect," including triggering any form of cancer, says CDC scientist Antonia Calafat, PhD. Still, because the health effects of everyday exposure to oxybenzone are unknown, experts believe more research is needed.

The bottom line: No studies prove, or even strongly suggest, that oxybenzone causes cancer. What is proven: Sunscreens are one of the best ways to protect against UV damage.

"We know the benefits of using them," says Kenneth Portier, PhD, of the American Cancer Society. "We don't know that there's any harm." If the FDA becomes aware of information indicating that any sunscreens are unsafe, it says it will warn the public. Still concerned? Opt for one that doesn't have oxybenzone.

Concern: Tiny particles may get into skin and trigger health problems

Background: If you use sunscreen geared for sensitive skin, it probably contains titanium dioxide and zinc oxide. These ingredients work by reflecting—instead of absorbing—UV rays, so they tend to be less irritating. In their regular form, both are made up of large particles that leave a white film on skin—think of the thick white coating you used to see on a lifeguard's nose.

To make sunscreens more transparent and less like clown makeup, titanium and zinc are now often engineered into ultrasmall nanoparticles. (As a bonus, they fit better into the nooks and crannies of the skin to create more even coverage.) The problem: No one really knew whether these tiny particles could penetrate skin and build up in the body—and if they did, whether that was dangerous. (One theory is that they might get into cells and cause DNA damage.)

Turns out this worry about nanos might have been for naught, as a growing body of research—including two studies published earlier this year, one by FDA scientists—shows these particles don't absorb through healthy or damaged skin.

One still unanswered question is whether nanoparticles trigger free radicals when exposed to UV light. Manufacturers can squelch their production with a specific form of titanium dioxide, but a recent study suggests that some of them may not be using it. Unless the FDA mandates its use, consumers can't know for sure if it's in their sunscreen.

The bottom line: "It's virtually impossible to prove something is completely safe no matter how many studies are done, but the weight of evidence suggests that nanoparticles in sunscreens won't present a risk to your health," says Andrew Maynard, PhD, director of the University of Michigan Risk Science Center. Even the EWG now recommends these sunscreens as "among the safest, most effective on the market."

Concern: Sunscreen blocks production of vitamin D

Background: Though an SPF 30 sunscreen blocks 97 percent of UVB, the rays that enable skin to create vitamin D, research shows that normal use

SAFE SUNSCREENS THAT BLOCK WELL, TOO

Whatever your needs, each of these five products provides strong UVA protection.

BEST FOR SENSITIVE SKIN: Coppertone Sensitive Skin Sunscreen Lotion improved redness and broken capillaries after 4 weeks in one study ($10; drugstores).*

BEST MOISTURIZER WITH SPF: Vichy Aqualia Thermal Lotion SPF 30 24 Hr Hydrating Moisturizer saves you a step in the morning ($28; drugstores).

BEST AGE-ERASING BLOCK: Neutrogena Age Shield + Repair Anti-Aging Sunblock SPF 55 ($10; drugstores) packs soy to fade brown spots.**

BEST FOR MIDDAY TOUCH-UPS: Colorescience Pro Sunforgettable Mineral Powder Sun Protection SPF 50, a brush-on sunscreen, goes on slightly tinted so you don't miss spots—but the color quickly fades to match all skin tones ($60; www.colorescience.com).

BEST FOR ACNE-PRONE SKIN: Bullfrog Quik Gel Sport Spray SPF 50 is oil-free and won't clog pores ($10; drugstores).**

*contains nanoparticles

**contains oxybenzone

doesn't generally result in vitamin D deficiency—in part because few of us apply (or reapply) enough. Still, with its growing reputation as a wonder vitamin, D is one nutrient you don't want to be lacking in. Studies indicate many people are.

The bottom line: The simplest solution is to get more D into your diet (good sources include salmon, cheese, and fortified milk and juice), and take a daily supplement of 1,000 IU of vitamin D3.

"It's so easy and a whole lot safer than frying your skin in the sun," says James Spencer, MD, a clinical professor of dermatology at Mount Sinai School of Medicine.

ANSWER KEY for Chapter 24

Here are the answers to the brain games.

WEEK 1 DAY 4—FIND IT (FROM LEFT): 14, 18, 14 (page 269)

WEEK 1 DAY 6—GET THE PICTURE: large window, blinds on large window, white sofa, white ottoman, 2 striped pillows, gold pillow, burgundy pillow, floor plant, coffee table, lamp on coffee table, wooden object on coffee table, small violin, 3 small windows, bookshelf, books, globe, small plant on bookshelf, small lamp on bookshelf, vase on bookshelf, bowl on bookshelf, beige carpet (page 269)

WEEK 3 DAY 3—REBUS RALLY: 1. Big bad wolf 2. Slow down 3. Read between the lines 4. Eggs over easy 5. Keep in touch 6. Scotch on the rocks (page 278)

WEEK 4 DAY 1—TRIANGLES: 13 (page 279)

WEEK 4 DAY 7—DECODE THIS: Brain training is fun (page 281)

PHOTO CREDITS

Pages 89-91, 104-105 ©Shay Peretz

Pages 98-102 ©Karen Pearson

Page 151 ©Melanie Grizzel

Pages 162-163 ©Alexa Miller

Pages 168-171 ©Christa Renee

Pages 177-180 ©Shannon Greer

Pages 191-195 ©Saye

Page 201 ©Anna Knot

Page 257 ©Taghi Naderzad

Pages 269, 271-273, 278-281 ©Headcase Design

Page 270 ©iStockPhoto

Pages 286-289 ©Justin Steele

INDEX

Boldface page references indicate photographs and illustrations. Underscored references indicate boxed text.

Body fat
   abdominal, 23
   workout for losing, 157–59, 161, <u>161</u>
Body mass index, 23
Bone health
   calcium for, <u>26</u>, 245
   cauliflower for, <u>209</u>
   pasta with parsley for, 211
   vitamin D for, <u>26</u>, 245, <u>317</u>
   vitamin K for, <u>209</u>
Botox, 307
Bowling, calories burned by, <u>110</u>
Brain health. *See* Mental health
Brainpower Game Plan
   overview, 268
   Week 1, 268–70, **269**
   Week 2, 270–73, **271**, **272**, **273**
   Week 3, 276–81, **279**
   Week 4, 279–81, **281**
BRCA 1 or 2 gene, 30
Breads and bread crumbs
   Berry Good Peanut Butter Scones,
      123
   Chocolate-Stuffed French Toast, 121
   Cod Cakes, 144
   Easy Barbecue Pita Pizzas, 128
   Lemon-Blueberry Buttermilk
      Muffins, 124
   Pistachio Cheese Spread, 129
   Tomato-Topped Meat Loaf, 141
   Tomato and Roasted Pepper
      Bruschetta, 127
   as weight loss aid, <u>78</u>
   Whole Grain Stuffing with
      Sausage, 136
Breakfast
   benefit of, 63
   Berry Good Peanut Better Scones,
      123

Chocolate-Stuffed French Toast,
   121
Lemon-Blueberry Buttermilk
   Muffins, 124
More-Vegetable-Than-Egg
   Frittata, 120
Walnut-Pear Pancake with Maple
   Syrup, 122
weight loss and, <u>66</u>
Breast cancer, 26, <u>236</u>, 347
Broccoli, <u>212</u>
Broth, <u>181</u>
Brown sugar
   antioxidants in, <u>225</u>
   Berry Good Peanut Butter Scones,
      123
   Orange-Glazed Ham, 143
   as sweetener, <u>225</u>
Bruises, healing, 208
Brushing teeth, <u>275</u>. *See also* Oral
   health
Brussels sprouts, <u>214</u>
Buffet eating guidelines, <u>69</u>
B vitamins, <u>214–15</u>, <u>316</u>, 331

C

Caesar dressing, 74
Caffeine, 330
CAFOs, 253–54
Calcium
   for bone health, <u>26</u>, 245
   in cheese, <u>80</u>
   in nonfat powdered milk, 210
Calories
   in beverages, <u>62</u>, <u>66</u>
   burning, <u>110</u>
   exercises burning, <u>172</u>
   in high fructose corn syrup, 224
   longevity and intake of, 21

Vitamin B$_{12}$ deficiency, <u>316</u>

Vitamin C
    in bell peppers, 208
    in carrots, <u>212</u>
    in jicama, <u>209</u>
    in parsnips, <u>209</u>
    in radishes, <u>209</u>
    in skin care, 14, 322
    in sunscreen, 347
    in wrinkle prevention, 14

Vitamin D
    balance and, <u>27</u>
    for bone health, <u>26</u>, 245, <u>317</u>
    deficiency, 349
    in farmed salmon, lack of, <u>230</u>
    in nonfat powered milk, 210
    sunscreen and absorption of,
        348–49
    supplements, <u>26</u>

Vitamin E, 208, 243–44, 322–23,
    347

Vitamin K, <u>209</u>, 211, 323

Vitamins. *See specific type*

W

Waist measurement, 23

Wakeup time, <u>298</u>

Walking
    for energy, <u>284</u>
    pedometer with, 17
    with poles, <u>173</u>
    program
        8-week plan, 84–87, <u>85</u>
        body-sculpting exercises, <u>86</u>, 87,
            89–91, **89–91**
        experts advising on, <u>86</u>
        marathon, 88, 91–93, <u>92–93</u>
        strategies for sticking with, <u>85</u>

weight loss and, 83–84
in winter, <u>115</u>

Walnuts
    antioxidants in, <u>276</u>
    for mental health, <u>276</u>
    Roasted Beet Salad, 131
    Walnut-Pear Pancake with Maple
        Syrup, 122

Warfarin (Coumadin), 4–5, <u>32–33</u>

Water intake, 198

Weight loss. *See also* Food,
        substitutes; Workouts
    aging and, 175
    benefits of, 61–62
    breakfast and, <u>66</u>
    buffet eating guidelines and, <u>69</u>
    cardio exercise and, <u>160</u>
    depression prevention and, 62
    fiber and, <u>68</u>
    foods aiding, <u>78–81</u>
    goals, 69–70
    headache prevention and, 61
    journals
        Benavides, Melissa, 151–53, **151**
        Montague, Sarah, 201–3, **201**
    oral health and, 62
    plateau busters
        Brennan, Chrissy, 108–10
        Coulson, Donna, 110–12
        experts advising on, 107, <u>108</u>
        Spodak, Lisa, 112–14
    running and, 190
    saboteurs
        assuming calories from healthy,
            natural foods are low, 68
        dieting issues, <u>64–67</u>
        eating like a bird for the month
            leading up to a big event, 68–69